The Brompton Hospital
Guide to
Chest Physiotherapy

Compiled by
D. V. Gaskell MCSP
and
B. A. Webber MCSP

The Brompton
Hospital Guide to
Chest Physiotherapy

Second edition, third printing

Blackwell Scientific Publications

OXFORD LONDON EDINBURGH MELBOURNE

Published by Blackwell Scientific Publications
Osney Mead, Oxford, England
85 Marylebone High Street, London W1, England
9 Forrest Road, Edinburgh, Scotland
P.O. Box 9, North Balwyn, Victoria, Australia

ISBN 0 632 09670 5

First published 1960
Revised reprints 1962, 1964, 1967
Second edition 1973
Revised reprint 1974
Reprinted 1975

Distributed in the U.S.A. by
J. B. Lippincott Company, Philadelphia
and in Canada by
J. B. Lippincott Company of
Canada Ltd, Toronto

Printed and bound in Great Britain by
Billing & Sons Limited,
Guildford and London

Contents

Preface

This book is intended as a practical guide for physiotherapists and others concerned with the treatment of chest conditions. It is derived from the booklet *Physiotherapy for Medical and Surgical Thoracic Conditions* originally compiled at the Brompton Hospital in 1960.

The development of physiotherapeutic techniques in the treatment of chest disease was begun at the Brompton Hospital in 1934 by the late Miss Winifred Linton, FCSP(HON), who became superintendent physiotherapist at that time. These techniques have subsequently been further developed and modified as advances in the medical and surgical management of chest disease have occurred, and more understanding of the physiology of normal respiration has been gained.

The basic techniques of breathing exercises, and postural drainage and an outline of the relevant anatomy are described. Physiotherapy for a wide variety of medical and surgical cardio-thoracic conditions is included. There are also sections on the treatment of patients undergoing artificial ventilation and an account of the uses of inter-mittent positive pressure breathing as a valuable adjunct to physiotherapy.

In order to make intelligent use of the techniques described in the following text, the physiotherapist must have a detailed knowledge of the anatomical mechanism of respiration and the physiology of gaseous exchange. A basic knowledge of the interpretation of electrocardiographs is also useful. This additional knowledge can be obtained from the appropriate text books.

It is important to appreciate that the physiotherapist is a member of a team which includes nurses, technicians and the patient, all under the direction of a physician or surgeon. The more each person is cognisant of the others' contribution, and the more their efforts are co-ordinated, the better will be the results.

The authors would like to thank Dr M.A.Branthwaite, MRCP, FFARCS, for assistance and advice given during the preparation of this book. They are also grateful to Professor R.J.Last, FRCS, and to Mrs S.A.Hyde, MCSP, for their helpful suggestions.

D.V.G.
B.A.W.

1 Anatomy of the thoracic cage and lungs

Movements of the rib cage

An understanding of the normal mechanism of respiration is essential before teaching breathing exercises. This mechanism depends not only on the anatomy of the respiratory muscles, but in particular the ribs and their articulations in the thoracic cage. To quote Professor R.J.Last: 'The ribs are to breathe with.'

During respiration, changes in volume of the thoracic cage are brought about in three diameters.

The antero-posterior diameter of the thorax is increased by elevation of the ribs. The manubrium of the sternum is fixed by a primary cartilaginous joint to the first costal cartilage, and the manubrium and the first ribs are fixed to each other and move together as one. As the manubrium is elevated its lower border projects anteriorly. This border articulates by a hinge joint to the body of the sternum, movement occurring at this joint as the body of the sternum rises with the ribs. (If this joint becomes ankylosed, thoracic expansion is virtually lost.)

The costal cartilages of the second to seventh ribs articulate with the sternum by a synovial joint, and the eighth, ninth and tenth costal cartilages articulate with the cartilage above by a synovial joint.

The ribs slope downwards from their attachment to the vertebral column towards the sternum, at an angle of 45°. Rotation of the neck of the ribs occurs at all twelve costo-vertebral joints and this results in elevation or depression of the anterior ends of the ribs.

As a result of the obliquity of the ribs,

elevation of the sternum carries it forwards and thus the antero-posterior diameter of the thorax is increased. This up and down movement of the body of the sternum, and the ribs attached to it, is often termed the 'pump-handle movement'.

The transverse diameter of the thorax is increased in two ways, one passive and the other active. The passive increase is due to the shape of the ribs and the axis round which they hinge during inspiration. The axis is not transverse across the body, but passes through the head and tubercle of

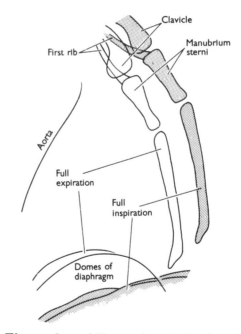

Fig. 1. *Lateral X-ray view of the thoracic cavity of a healthy young male, showing maximum excursion simultaneously of the chest wall and of the diaphragm. From R.J.Last* Anatomy, Regional and Applied, *5th edition, Churchill.*

I

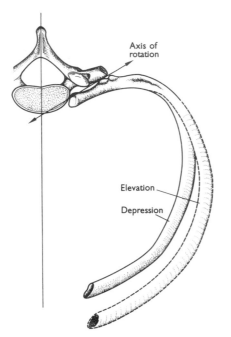

Axis of rotation

Elevation

Depression

Fig. 2. *The axis of rotation of a rib. From R.J.Last* Anatomy, Regional and Applied, *5th edition, Churchill.*

each rib obliquely backwards from the mid-line (figs. 1 & 2). Therefore the downward sloping rib is not only elevated antero-posteriorly but also laterally. This lateral spread of the ribs increases from the fifth rib downwards because the costal cartilages become progressively more oblique. It does not occur in the upper four pairs, as their costal cartilages are too short to allow such separation from the mid line.

The active increase in transverse diameter is brought about by the 'bucket-handle' movement of the lower ribs. These ribs rotate about an axis that passes through the anterior and posterior extremity of each, like lifting up the fallen handle from the side of a bucket.

This movement can occur because the articular surfaces of the seventh to tenth costo-vertebral joints are flat; the tubercles of these ribs can move up and down, in addition to the rotation occurring at the neck of the rib.

The vertical diameter of the thorax is increased by descent of the diaphragm.

The muscles of inspiration

The most important muscle of inspiration is the diaphragm. It is a bi-domed muscle, its fibres originating from the sternum, the lower ribs and the upper lumbar vertebrae. In full expiration the right dome rises to the level of the 4th intercostal space (nipple level), while the left dome is at the level of the 5th rib. The central tendon is level with the lower end of the sternum. In quiet inspiration, only the domes of the diaphragm descend and there is no movement of the central tendon. In a deeper breath, further descent of the domes below the level of the central tendon can depress the central tendon from the level of the 8th thoracic vertebra to the 9th thoracic vertebra. This stretches the mediastinum and no further descent of the central tendon is possible. The diaphragm will only descend if the abdominal wall relaxes. With further contraction of the muscle (i.e. maximum inspiration) the outer fibres evert the ribs of the costal margin in the 'bucket-handle' movement.

The 12th rib, held down by quadratus lumborum, is not elevated with the other ribs. This fixes the posterior fibres of the diaphragm and increases the vertical diameter of the thorax.

The fibres of the external intercostal muscles pass obliquely downwards and forwards between the ribs. When the muscles contract, they lift the ribs in a powerful inspiratory movement. The external intercostal muscle fibres cease and become a membrane between the costal cartilages. These cartilages slope in the opposite obliquity to the ribs, and the part of the internal intercostal muscle that lies between these costal cartilages elevates them when its fibres shorten.

The accessory muscles of inspiration can be brought into action to produce an increase in ventilation. The sternomastoids, with the help of the scalene muscles, elevate the thoracic inlet, while the head extensor muscles fix the head in extension. If the arms are fixed in abduction, the muscles attaching the upper limbs to the trunk are inspiratory; these are the pectoral muscles, serratus anterior, and the costal fibres of latissimus dorsi.

The muscles of expiration

During quiet or forced expiration the diaphragm is completely passive, its relaxed fibres being elongated by pressure from below.

Depression of the ribs and sternum is passive during quiet expiration. It is brought about by the elastic recoil of the chest wall and lungs. To produce a forced expiration the lateral fibres of the internal intercostal muscles contract, depressing the ribs. The thoracic cage is also depressed by the downward pull of the rectus abdominis and oblique abdominal muscles, on the ribs; at the same time the abdominal muscles elevate the diaphragm by raising the intra-abdominal pressure.

Structure of airways and alveoli

It is not intended to give a detailed description of the anatomy and physiology of the respiratory system, but a few facts con-

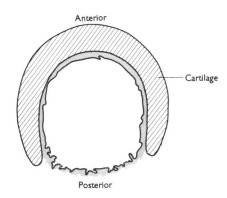

Fig. 3. *Trachea during normal breathing.*

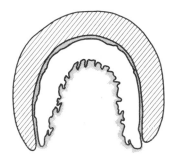

Fig. 4. *Trachea during cough—internal area reduced to ⅙ of its normal area.*

cerning the structure of the airways are described to assist the understanding of some mechanisms involved in respiratory physiotherapy.

The *trachea* extends from the cricoid cartilage (lower border of C6) to the bifurcation of the main bronchi at the level of the angle of Louis (upper border of T5). It is lined by ciliated columnar epithelium containing plentiful mucus-secreting glands and goblet cells. The wall is a fibro-elastic membrane whose patency is maintained by C-shaped rings of cartilage. The gaps lie posteriorly and are closed by a sheet of muscle which plays an important part in the efficacy of coughing.

To produce a *cough*, a forced expiratory

3

effort is made against a closed **glottis** causing a rise in intrathoracic pressure. The glottis then opens abruptly so that a large pressure gradient exists between the alveolar pressure and the upper tracheal pressure (now atmospheric). A very rapid flow rate results. The high intrathoracic pressure inverts the posterior non-cartilaginous part of the intrathoracic trachea and narrows it to one sixth of its normal area (figs. 3 & 4). The rapid flow rate combined with this narrowing increases the explosive force of the air which dislodges mucus and foreign particles, bringing them to the pharynx.

The *bronchi* are airways which have cartilage in their walls. The proximal five generations have abundant cartilage, but the fifth to fifteenth generations are smaller bronchi with scattered plates of cartilage throughout the walls. The walls of the bronchi also contain fibrous tissue with a capillary network, and longitudinal bands of elastic fibres. They are lined by layers of ciliated epithelium containing numerous mucus-secreting glands and goblet cells.

Bronchioli are airways distal to the last plate of cartilage and proximal to the alveolar region. They are about 1 mm or less in diameter. Their walls are composed of smooth muscle fibres arranged circularly, and lined by epithelium containing some mucous glands and goblet cells. The distal bronchioli are lined with only one layer of epithelium and have very few mucus-secreting cells.

In massive collapse of a lobe the large bronchi are inherently rigid enough to remain patent, whereas the walls of the small bronchi and bronchioli collapse and come into apposition.

All bronchioli eventually reach a point where alveoli open into the lumen. This part is known as the *respiratory bronchiole*.

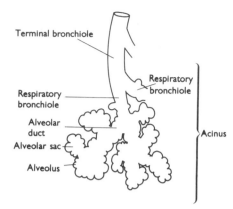

Fig. 5. *Respiratory bronchiole.*

A *terminal bronchiole* is defined as the airway immediately proximal to the respiratory bronchiole (fig. 5). The terminal bronchioli contain no cilia and no mucus-secreting glands or goblet cells.

An *acinus* is the area of lung distal to the terminal bronchiole, and includes several generations of respiratory bronchioli (up to 8), alveolar ducts, and alveoli. An acinus is approximately 0·5–1 cm in diameter.

A recent estimate of the total number of alveoli in the average adult lung is thought to be in the region of 300 million.

An *alveolus* is an air sac consisting of a single layer of flat cells and a network of fine elastic fibres. A rich network of capillaries surrounds it.

Alveolar pores are openings that exist in the alveolar walls of the human lung allowing drift of air from alveolus to alveolus, and thereby from lobule to lobule and segment to segment, without using the airways. This phenomenon is known as *collateral air drift*, and by providing alternative pathways for the passage of air, collapse of segments of a lung distal to a plugged bronchus does not necessarily occur. The pleura prevents drift of air between the lobes of the lungs.

2 Breathing exercises and postural drainage

BREATHING EXERCISES

Aims

To obtain the best possible lung function by:
1 Promoting a normal relaxed pattern of breathing, where possible.
2 Teaching controlled breathing with the minimum amount of effort.
3 Assisting with removal of secretions.
4 Aiding re-expansion of lung tissue.
5 Mobilising the thoracic cage.

Practice

The necessity for frequent and regular practice must be emphasised to all patients being taught breathing exercises. Efficient progress will not be made if the patient only does his exercises when the physiotherapist is present.

The patient should be advised to carry out each exercise 18–24 times, in groups of 6, with a short rest between each group to avoid hyperventilation. This should be repeated 2–5 times a day, according to the patient's condition.

DIAPHRAGMATIC BREATHING

The term 'diaphragmatic breathing' is misleading since the diaphragm also plays an important part in lower costal expansion. Perhaps breathing control by correct use of the diaphragm would more accurately describe the following technique, but throughout the text 'diaphragmatic breathing' is used for want of a more concise term.

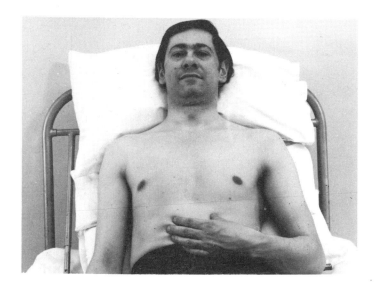

Fig. 6. *Diaphragmatic breathing*.

To teach diaphragmatic breathing the patient should be positioned so that his back and head are fully supported and his abdominal wall relaxed. If he is in bed, he should sit as high as possible with his knees slightly bent, or if he is out of bed, a high backed chair without arms is most suitable. The physiotherapist's hands rest lightly on the anterior costal margins to stimulate and palpate the movement occurring; later the patient is instructed to feel the movement himself (fig. 6).

He breathes out as quietly as possible, while relaxing the shoulders and chest and sinking the lower ribs down and in towards the mid-line. He is then told to breathe in gently and to 'feel the air coming in round his waist'. The upper chest and shoulders remain relaxed throughout. The emphasis is on gentle breathing with the minimum of effort. Once the patient has mastered this type of breathing it can be used with effect during attacks of dyspnoea, to improve ventilation and also to loosen secretions in the bases of the lungs.

The patient is closely observed during the training period so that the following common faults may be avoided:

1 *Forced expiration.* Expiration must be completely passive; it is vital to remember that any forcing or prolongation of expiration will tend to increase airways obstruction. In normal expiration the airways shorten and become narrower; therefore if the airways are already partially obstructed and the patient forces expiration, the flow of air will be further impeded. Forced expiration produces a rise in intrapleural pressure; air trapping may result if damaged collapsible airways are compressed by a rise in intrapleural pressure. Forced expiration ('huffing') is only of value in the removal of secretions in post-operative patients (p. 41).

2 *Prolonged expiration.* Patients should not be encouraged to attempt to empty their lungs completely. Respiration which follows will be irregular and inefficient.

3 *Trick movements* of the abdomen. The abdominal musculature may be contracted and relaxed without any resultant effect on ventilation.

4 *Over use of the upper chest* and accessory muscles are discouraged, as this can inhibit movement of the diaphragm.

LOCALISED EXPANSION EXERCISES

Although it is doubtful whether localised breathing exercises ventilate isolated lobes of the lung, they are useful for improving movement of the thoracic cage and for assisting the removal of secretions.

Pressure is applied to appropriate areas of the chest wall; utilising proprioceptive stimuli, more efficient expansion of these areas may be obtained. The patient should be in a half-lying position with the knees slightly flexed over a pillow, or where possible sitting on an upright chair or stool. The physiotherapist should position herself so that she can compare the movement of the two sides of the chest. Later, some of these exercises can be practised sitting in front of a mirror.

(a) Unilateral basal expansion

Unilateral basal expansion is thought to make use of the 'bucket handle' movement of the ribs, thus increasing the contraction of the outer fibres of the diaphragm.

The physiotherapist places the palm of her hand well round to the side in the mid-axillary line over the 7th, 8th and 9th ribs. The patient should be instructed to relax and breathe out, and feel the lower ribs sinking down and in; this movement should not be forced. At the end of expiration, the physiotherapist should apply firm pressure to the area described. The patient should be instructed with the next inspiration both to expand the lower ribs against her hand, and to direct the inspired air to that lung base. The pressure should not be excessive, as this could restrict rather than assist the movement. At full inspiration the pressure is released, and not reapplied until just before the patient is ready to breathe in again.

When the patient understands the localised movement required, he is taught to apply the pressure himself. This can be done in one of the following ways:

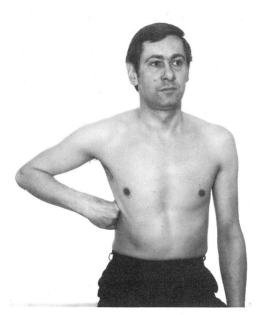

Fig. 7. *Unilateral basal expansion.*

1 With the palm of the hand placed well back in the mid-axillary line. If wrist extension is limited this method is unsuitable.
2 With the back of the fingers; the wrist being held in the mid-position or slight flexion (fig. 7).
3 With the palm of the opposite hand.

Any simulation of costal expansion by side-flexion of the spine should be recognised and corrected, and the patient should not be allowed to elevate his shoulder girdle when positioning his hands.

Many patients with obstructive airways disease must first achieve quiet expiration with relaxation of the over-inflated thoracic cage before they attempt basal expansion. The emphasis in surgical patients should be on the inspiratory phase; holding the maximum inspiration for one or two seconds is helpful. This will assist aeration of the peripheral alveoli by promoting the expansion of areas of poor compliance.

(b) Bilateral basal expansion

It is not advisable to use bilateral basal expansion for the 'upper chest breather', but with post-operative patients this can be a useful progression of treatment.

Pressure is applied in the mid-axillary line to both sides of the lower chest with the palms or backs of the hands. The exercise is carried out in exactly the same way as for unilateral expansion, but if the patient is applying his own pressure he often finds difficulty in relaxing the shoulder girdle adequately.

(c) Apical expansion (fig. 8)

This is useful when there is restricted upper chest movement, or incomplete expansion of lung tissue, particularly where there is an

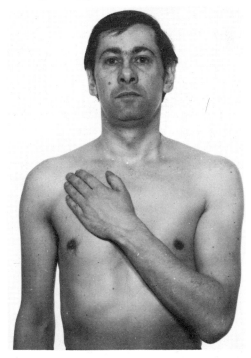

Fig. 8. *Apical expansion.*

apical pneumothorax, e.g. following lobectomy.

Pressure is applied below the clavicle using the tips of the fingers. The patient breathes in, expanding the chest forwards and upwards against the pressure of the fingers. The shoulders should be relaxed, and the expansion held momentarily before expiration. If the patient finds this exercise difficult he is instructed to hold his breath for a moment on full inspiration, and then to sniff two or three times before breathing out.

Occasionally, the following exercises may be helpful when the physiotherapist is trying to localise chest movement still further, but they are rarely used.

(d) Upper lateral expansion

The pressure is applied just below the axilla. The technique used is similar to that for unilateral basal expansion (p. 6).

(e) Posterior basal expansion

The patient, who should be sitting, leans forward from the hips with a straight back, and pressure is given unilaterally over the posterior aspect of the lower ribs. He can be taught to give this pressure himself.

BELT EXERCISES

When the physiotherapist is satisfied that the patient can localise his chest movement to some extent, it may be helpful for him to apply his own resistance, using a belt. By this method it is possible to relax the shoulder girdle more effectively, and many

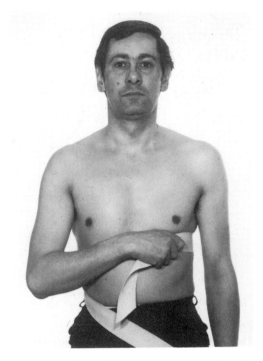

Fig. 9. *Unilateral basal expansion with belt.*

patients practise more conscientiously when a piece of equipment is involved.

Upholstery webbing makes suitable belts for this purpose. The width should be 2 in–2½ in (5–7 cm), and the length about 6 feet (2 metres) according to the patient's size.

The patient should be seated on a stool or upright chair, and it is often helpful to use a mirror.

(a) Unilateral basal expansion (fig. 9)

For the left side: the belt is placed round the lower chest at the level of the xiphisternum, with a short piece round the left side and held in front with the right hand. The right forearm should be pronated and the wrist in the mid-line so that the arm is in a relaxed

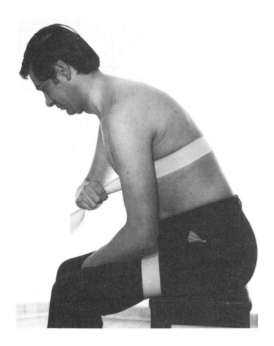

Fig. 10. *Posterior basal expansion with belt.*

(c) Posterior basal expansion (fig. 10)

The patient should sit leaning forward from the hips with a straight back. For the left side: the belt is placed round the back of the chest at the level of the xiphisternum. The piece of belt coming round from the left side is held forwards with the right hand in order to give pressure to the posterior part of the ribs. The other end of the belt is crossed over the thighs and is fixed under the left thigh. At the end of the breath out the patient pulls the belt firmly forwards, and he then breathes in and expands the ribs backwards against the resistance of the belt. At full inspiration the pressure is released and expansion is maintained for a moment before expiration.

The procedure is reversed for the right side.

position. The other end is crossed over the thighs and fixed under the left thigh. At the end of the breath out the patient pulls the belt firmly; he then breathes in and expands the left side of the chest outwards against the resistance of the belt. At full inspiration the pressure is released and expansion is maintained for a moment before expiration.

The procedure is reversed for the right side.

(b) Upper lateral expansion

If there is any indication for lateral expansion of the upper chest, a belt can be used in the same manner as for the previous exercise but it should be placed not more than 2 in (5 cm) below the axilla.

POSTURAL DRAINAGE

The patient is positioned to assist the drainage of secretions from specific areas of the lungs by means of gravity. The positions are based on the anatomy of the bronchial tree as shown in the diagrams (fig. 11). This drainage should be assisted by vibratory shaking or percussion of the chest, combined with localised breathing exercises. Where difficulty is experienced in expectoration (e.g. cystic fibrosis, asthma, infants with bronchiolitis), increased humidity may help.

The appropriate positions should be maintained for up to half an hour 2–6 times a day, according to the individual patient's needs. Ideally, a patient should remain in any one position until that particular area is clear of secretions, but sometimes he may

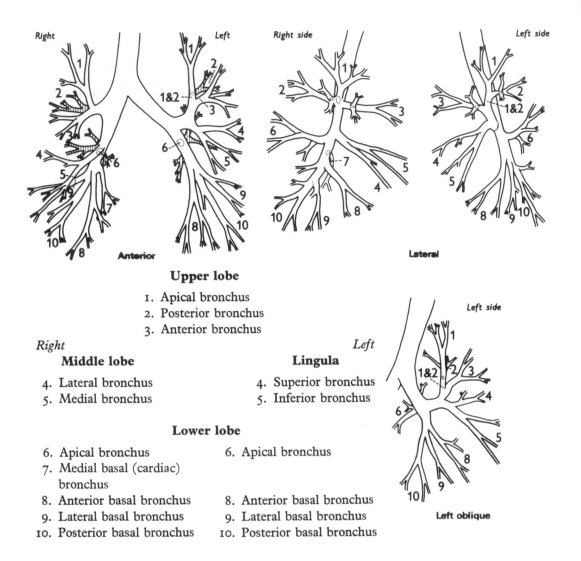

Upper lobe

1. Apical bronchus
2. Posterior bronchus
3. Anterior bronchus

Right   *Left*

Middle lobe   **Lingula**

4. Lateral bronchus   4. Superior bronchus
5. Medial bronchus   5. Inferior bronchus

Lower lobe

6. Apical bronchus   6. Apical bronchus
7. Medial basal (cardiac)
   bronchus
8. Anterior basal bronchus   8. Anterior basal bronchus
9. Lateral basal bronchus   9. Lateral basal bronchus
10. Posterior basal bronchus   10. Posterior basal bronchus

Fig. 11. *Diagram illustrating the broncho-pulmonary nomenclature approved by the Thoracic Society. Reproduced by permission of the Editors of* Thorax.

be unable to tolerate this. If the physio-therapist has to leave the patient in a drainage position, she should instruct him to practise expansion exercises and to cough at approximately 5-minute intervals, so that any secretions loosened by the treatment may be removed from the bronchial tree, and not be transferred to another area. The treatment will be inadequate if the patient is allowed to lie passively.

Instruction should be given in effective coughing. It is important to take a deep breath before coughing, and to contract the abdominal muscles during the cough. After two or three coughs, another deep breath should be taken; the patient should not be allowed to go into an uncontrolled paroxysm of coughing as this is ineffective and exhausting. If the patient persists in coughing without breathing in, cough syncope occasionally occurs.

It is inadvisable to carry out postural drainage immediately after a meal, as the patient may be induced to vomit, or at least feel nauseated, and will not perform the treatment adequately. Postural drainage is also unsuitable immediately before a meal, since the patient may have become too exhausted to enjoy his food. Some patients find it easier to cough productively after having a warm drink.

It is not always the postural drainage itself that gives most benefit to the patient; the breathing exercises, shaking and effective coughing are often the most important part of the treatment, particularly if the secretions are thick and tenacious.

Modified postural drainage

Some patients cannot lie flat without becoming dyspnoeic; this is known as orthopnoea. If a patient has secretions at the lung bases, and is likely to become distressed by orthodox postural drainage, it is better to compromise and lay him as flat as possible for short periods, on alternate sides, without tipping the bed. In this position, shaking and percussion may be given as usual. If this position does not cause distress, it may be taken a stage further by placing one or two pillows under the patient's hips in order to tilt his chest.

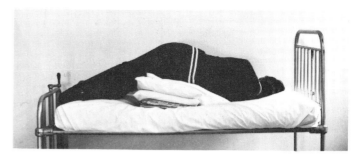

Fig. 12. *Position for postural drainage at home.*

Postural drainage at home

This can often present a problem, as it is difficult for the majority of patients to tip their bed at home. It can be overcome by placing a 6 in (15 cm) thick pile of newspapers or magazines, tied tightly together, in the centre of the bed with two pillows on top (fig. 12). The patient can lie over this in varying positions and thus drain most areas of the lungs.

Alternatively, a firm wedge of polyether foam can be obtained, but this is only suitable for children and light adults.

Other methods can be evolved by the ingenuity of the physiotherapist and the patient, making use of the furniture in the home (e.g. using an upturned chair).

These methods may not provide an efficient enough tipping position for certain patients suffering from severe basal bronchiectasis or cystic fibrosis. It is important to find some means of tipping the bed, or for patients with insurmountable problems it might be necessary to arrange for the loan of a hospital tipping bed. The deep tipping position that is sometimes used with a patient lying over the side of the bed, is rarely suitable. Most patients find it un-

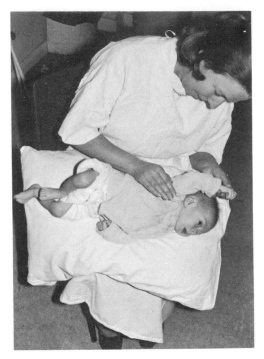

Fig. 13. *Postural drainage for a baby. By permission of Cystic Fibrosis Research Trust.*

comfortable, and it is only possible to drain the posterior basal segments of the lower lobes in this position.

Small children and infants can be given postural drainage by placing them over the knee (fig. 13); in the latter case it is usually most convenient to do this immediately prior to a feed.

Before a patient is discharged from hospital, he should be shown how to carry out appropriate postural drainage at home. The time factor should be taken into consideration, as it is not always possible to spend as long on treatment at home as it is in hospital. The patient should be encouraged to drain for as long as is practicable, until most of the secretions have been cleared. This should be at least 15–20 minutes, twice daily in most cases.

Bronchography

If there appears to be an excessive quantity of secretions which could prevent adequate outlining of the bronchi by the contrast medium in a bronchogram, the patient should be given appropriate postural drainage before the procedure.

After a bronchogram most patients do not require postural drainage, as the majority of the contrast medium is sucked into the peripheral bronchi during inspiration, and is gradually absorbed into the blood stream. The small amount of the medium remaining in the upper airways is removed by the action of the cilia and a few effective coughs.

With bronchiectasis the contrast medium is unlikely to be sucked as far into the periphery owing to the blockage of the small airways with sputum. The cilia will probably have been destroyed in these bronchiectatic airways and postural drainage will speed up the procedure of clearing the bronchi, although the medium itself does no harm to the patient. These patients should be carrying out regular postural drainage in any case.

It is important that patients have nothing to eat or drink for at least four hours after a bronchogram, until the effect of the local anaesthetic has worn off.

Postural drainage positions (figs. 14–24)

LOBE		POSTURE
Upper Lobe	1. Apical bronchus	1. Sitting upright; with slight variations according to position of lesion, i.e. slightly leaning backwards, forwards or sideways.
	2. Posterior bronchus	
	(a) Right	2a. Lying on left side horizontally, and then turned 45° on to face, resting against a pillow, with another supporting the head.
	(b) Left	2b. Lying on right side turned 45° on to face, with 3 pillows arranged to lift shoulders 12 in (30 cm) from bed.
	3. Anterior bronchus	3. Lying flat on back with knees slightly flexed.
Middle Lobe	4. Lateral bronchus	4 & 5. Lying flat on back, body quarter turned to left maintained by a pillow under right side from shoulder to hip. Foot of bed raised 14 in (35 cm).
	5. Medial Bronchus	
Lingula	4. Superior bronchus	4 & 5. Lying flat on back, body quarter turned to right maintained by a pillow under left side from shoulder to hip. Foot of bed raised 14 in (35 cm).
	5. Inferior bronchus	
Lower Lobe	6. Apical bronchus	6. Lying flat on face, pillow under the hips.
	7. Medial basal (Cardiac) bronchus	7. Lying on right side with a pillow under the hips, foot of bed raised 18 in (45 cm).
	8. Anterior basal bronchus	8. Lying flat on back, buttocks resting on a pillow and knees flexed, foot of bed raised 18 in (45 cm).
	9. Lateral basal bronchus	9. Lying on opposite side, foot of bed raised 18 in (45 cm), a pillow under the hips.
	10. Posterior basal bronchus	10. Lying flat on face with a pillow under the hips, foot of bed raised 18 in (45 cm).

13

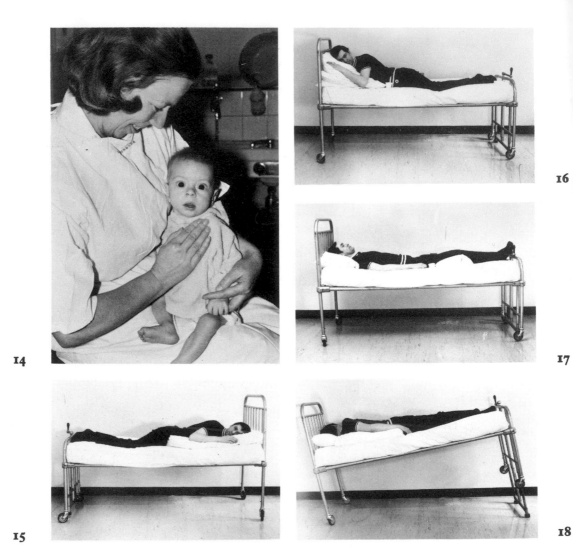

Fig. 14. *Apical segment, left upper lobe. By permission of Cystic Fibrosis Research Trust.*
Fig. 15. *Posterior segment, right upper lobe.*

Fig. 16. *Posterior segment, left upper lobe.*
Fig. 17. *Anterior segments, upper lobes.*
Fig. 18. *Right middle lobe.*

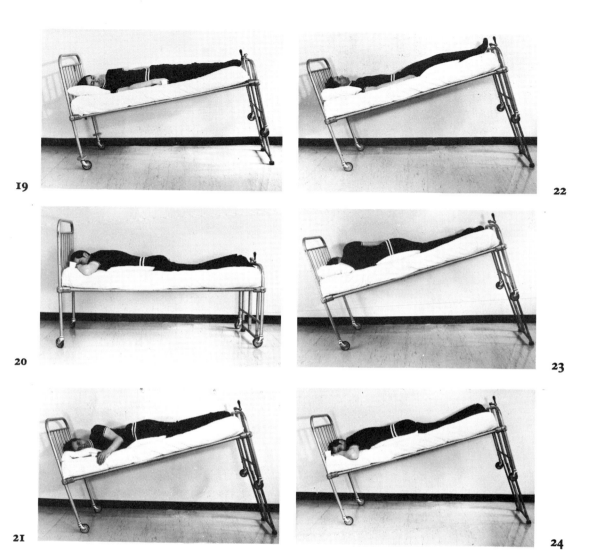

Fig. 19. *Lingula.*
Fig. 20. *Apical segments, lower lobes.*
Fig. 21. *Right medial basal and left lateral basal segments, lower lobes.*

Fig. 22. *Anterior basal segments, lower lobes.*
Fig. 23. *Lateral basal segment, right lower lobe.*
Fig. 24. *Posterior basal segments, lower lobes.*

3 Oxygen therapy

Oxygen therapy is often required in the management of patients with chest disease, but it is important to control the concentration of oxygen in some clinical circumstances.

An understanding of when oxygen must be prescribed with caution requires some knowledge of the normal chemical control of breathing.

In health, the level of the arterial carbon dioxide tension is the most important single factor controlling the rate and depth of breathing. A variety of mechanisms stimulate breathing when metabolic requirements are increased, as for example during exercise, and the level of carbon dioxide in the arterial blood remains surprisingly constant. An increase in this level beyond the normal range causes a sensation of severe breathlessness and stimulates the healthy person to hyperventilate vigorously, so removing the excess carbon dioxide and restoring the level to normal.

Some chronic lung diseases are characterised by the patient's tendency to breathe inadequately because the work of breathing is excessive and the efficiency of gas exchange is lowered by airway obstruction. A good example of such a condition is chronic bronchitis with secondary emphysema. If breathing is inadequate, the level of carbon dioxide in the blood tends to rise and the level of oxygen tends to fall. The respiratory centre slowly becomes acclimatised to the abnormally high level of carbon dioxide in the arterial blood and no longer responds by stimulating an increase in the rate and depth of breathing. When the respiratory centre no longer matches respiratory effort to the patient's requirements, the only stimulus which keeps the patient breathing regularly is the lack of oxygen (hypoxia) in the blood.

Hypoxia is dangerous because many organs, e.g. the heart and kidneys, suffer from oxygen lack. If hypoxia is relieved by the administration of high concentrations of oxygen, the last effective stimulus to respiration is removed and breathing becomes progressively more shallow and ineffective, so allowing the carbon dioxide level to rise even further. The elevated carbon dioxide level renders the patient drowsy and unco-operative and eventually comatose. He is unable to cough and secretions accumulate in the lungs so adding to his respiratory disability. The oxygen lack has been relieved so he retains a 'good' colour, and often looks unusually flushed and hot because of the effects of excess carbon dioxide on the skin. This condition is very dangerous and may be fatal.

Controlled oxygen therapy, the administration of *low* concentrations of oxygen (24–35%) will *partly* relieve the hypoxia, so reducing the risk of damage to the body, without completely eliminating the stimulus to breathe. The level of carbon dioxide may rise a little when even low concentrations of oxygen are used, but in many patients it is possible to reach an equilibrium position in which both carbon dioxide and oxygen levels in the blood are acceptable. This is best achieved by serial measurement of blood gas values; alternatively, the oxygen concentration may be increased *slowly* (over several hours) up to 28%, observing the patient for any deterioration in conscious level or ability to cough and co-operate. Any deterioration in the mental state indicates that excessive oxygen has been used, and the concentration must be readjusted. If a satisfactory position cannot be achieved or if serious hypoxia persists in spite of all attempts to remove secretions and relieve spasm, intubation and intermittent positive pressure ventilation (IPPV) are generally necessary.

Not all patients with chronic lung disease respond in this way. In acute asthma, the patient may even breathe more deeply or frequently than is necessary to maintain the normal level of carbon dioxide in the blood, in an attempt to relieve the hypoxia which is always a common feature of the condition.

In the older age groups, or those with chronic asthma, and in all patients when fatigued, this ability to hyperventilate is lost and inadequate ventilation and elevation of the carbon dioxide level in the blood may follow. Until this stage is reached, most patients with asthma benefit from oxygen in high concentrations.

In another group of disorders (pulmonary oedema, fibrosing alveolitis, sarcoidosis, and pulmonary embolism) the ability to absorb oxygen is impaired to a much greater degree than the ability to excrete carbon dioxide, largely because a considerable percentage of the pulmonary blood flows to parts of the lung which are not being properly ventilated and the 'good' areas of lung compensate for the 'bad' in terms of carbon dioxide removal but not for the uptake of oxygen. This is because of the different diffusing capacities of carbon dioxide and oxygen. These patients are always very breathless. They generally breathe more deeply and frequently than is

necessary to maintain a normal carbon dioxide level, in an attempt to relieve the hypoxia. They require oxygen in the highest possible concentration, and there is no risk of respiratory depression because the respiratory centre never loses its normal sensitivity to carbon dioxide.

Oxygen may be used to drive an intermittent positive pressure breathing apparatus for treatment in conjunction with physiotherapy. With many of these machines, the percentage of oxygen received by the patient will be considerably higher than the controlled percentage delivered by the appropriate Venturi mask (fig. 25), e.g. in the treatment of the chronic bronchitic. This higher percentage is rarely dangerous during treatment, provided IPPB is not being administered too frequently, because the patient's ventilation is assisted and the

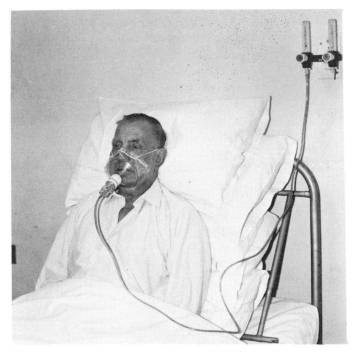

Fig. 25. *Venturi mask for oxygen therapy.*

17

removal of secretions from the chest as a result of treatment often leads to an improvement in the general condition. If however, the patient becomes more drowsy during or after treatment, the percentage of oxygen delivered by the machine is sometimes presumed to have been too high and therapy is prescribed with the machine driven by compressed air instead of oxygen. Ideally, an attachment to the machine should be available to provide a controlled quantity of added oxygen, while the machine is driven by compressed air.

Conversely, when treating patients with acute asthma, fibrosing alveolitis or left ventricular failure, etc., it is equally dangerous to use an IPPB machine driven entirely by compressed air. These patients need oxygen; the machine should either be driven by compressed oxygen or, again ideally, treatment should be carried out using a machine able to provide the optimal concentration of oxygen.

It is important to remember that oxygen is a drug and must, like all drugs, be carefully used so that undesirable side effects may be avoided. If a patient is receiving oxygen therapy, the mask should not be removed during breathing exercises, except for expectoration.

4   Medical conditions

TYPES OF DISABILITY

Two disorders characterise many medical chest diseases. Although these features are combined in many conditions, one of them usually predominates. The disorders are as follows:

1   Obstructive airways disease

The flow of air through the lungs may be reduced by obstruction in the airways. It can be assessed by measuring the FEV_1 (forced expiratory volume in 1 second) which is normally 70-80% of the FVC (forced vital capacity). The FVC and FEV_1 are recorded on machines which give a spirogram trace, such as the Vitalograph or Vitalor. Alternatively, the Peak Expiratory Flow Rate may be measured by means of the Wright Peak Flow Meter. This measures maximum flow over 10 milli-seconds at the beginning of expiration (fig. 26).

If the FEV_1 and PEFR improve following the administration of a bronchodilator the condition is recognised as *reversible airways obstruction* (fig. 27); this is frequently seen in asthma and chronic bronchitis. Reversible airways obstruction is caused by broncho-spasm, oedema of the bronchial mucosa or excessive secretions; a combination of all three is often present. These patients frequently respond well to a regime of bronchodilators and physiotherapy; some may require corticosteroids in addition.

If the FEV_1 and peak flow do not improve following administration of a bronchodilator, this is known as *irreversible airways obstruction*. It is a sign of structural damage of the

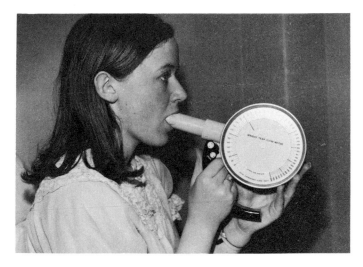

Fig. 26. *Peak flow meter in use.*

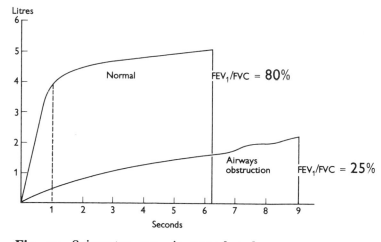

Fig. 27. *Spirometry.* FEV_1 *in normal and obstructed airways. By courtesy of Dr D.A.Ryland.*

19

airways and is seen in emphysema, severe chronic bronchitis and generalised bronchiectasis. These patients will only gain minimal improvement from drugs, but physiotherapy will be helpful with removal of secretions, and with teaching the patient a more co-ordinated pattern of breathing.

2 Restrictive pulmonary disease

Pulmonary expansion may be restricted by abnormalities of the rib cage, pleura or lungs.

Disorders of the rib cage include conditions such as ankylosing spondylitis and kyphoscoliosis. The flow of air in the lungs is reduced although there is no bronchial disease.

With disorders of the pleura or lungs, such as pleural fibrosis, interstitial pulmonary fibrosis (fibrosing alveolitis), or pulmonary oedema, there is a decrease in pulmonary compliance (increased stiffness) which restricts lung expansion.

The lung volumes are reduced in patients with restrictive lung disease, and to achieve adequate gaseous exchange breathing may be rapid (tachypnoea).

Diseases of the lung itself often interfere with the alveolar wall adding difficulties of gas transfer to those of pulmonary restriction.

OBSTRUCTIVE AIRWAYS DISEASES

This group of diseases includes chronic bronchitis, emphysema and asthma.

Assessment of the Patient

Before starting treatment, it is helpful to assess the condition of the patient.

Unless the patient is acutely ill, the physiotherapist should take a brief history before the first treatment. Simple lung function tests to measure the FEV$_1$ and FVC, or peak flow rate, are carried out to determine the degree of airways obstruction. Comparison with previous estimations is made where possible, to indicate the severity and nature of the condition, and the degree of reversibility which may be expected as a result of treatment.

Chest measurements are taken in order to assess chest movement, and repeated after a period of treatment to determine any improvement. The following method can be used, with the patient in the sitting position with his arms by his sides. Measurements are taken:

(i) As high in the axilla as possible; this is approximately at the level of the 4th rib.
(ii) In the epigastric region at about the level of the 9th costal cartilage. This is found by measuring three fingers breadth below the tip of the xiphoid process.
(iii) In the subcostal area, making certain that the tape measure is below the ribs.

The resting measurement is first noted. The tape measure is kept at the same tension round the chest, taking care not to draw it tight on expiration. The patient is instructed to breathe in fully, this measurement is not recorded; he should then breathe out completely and in again, these measurements being recorded, and the amount of expansion noted. The following is an example of a method of recording chest measurements.

Axilla (4th rib)

Resting	35 in	(89·5 cm)	
Expiration	34½ in	(88 cm)	} 2½ in
Inspiration	37 in	(94·5 cm)	} (6·5 cm)

Epigastrium

Resting	30 in	(76·5 cm)
Expiration	29½ in	(75·5 cm) ⎫ 1 in
Inspiration	30½ in	(78 cm) ⎭ (2·5 cm)

Subcostal

Resting	27 in	(69 cm)
Expiration	27 in	(69 cm) ⎫ ½ in
Inspiration	27½ in	(70·25 cm) ⎭ (1·25 cm)

When there is paradoxical movement of the chest wall, as in severe emphysema, the epigastric measurement may be greater on expiration and less on inspiration, the amount of expansion should be recorded with a minus, e.g. −½ in (−1·25 cm).

CHRONIC BRONCHITIS AND EMPHYSEMA

These two conditions were defined by the World Health Organisation in 1961 as follows:

Chronic bronchitis is a condition in which there is a chronic or recurrent increase above the normal in the volume of bronchial mucous secretion, sufficient to cause expectoration, when this condition is not due to localised broncho-pulmonary disease. The words 'chronic' or 'recurrent' may be further defined as present on most days during at least three months in each of two successive years.

Emphysema is a condition of the lung characterised by increase beyond the normal in the size of air spaces distal to the terminal bronchiole, with destructive changes in their walls.

Although these diseases have different pathological changes, each is characterised by airways obstruction and to some extent the principles underlying physiotherapy are similar.

The early chronic bronchitic will have hypertrophy of the mucous glands in the walls of the bronchi, and an increase of goblet cells in the epithelial lining of the bronchial tree. This causes excessive production of mucus which predisposes the patient to infection.

Repeated infections over the years will involve the alveoli in acute inflammation, and their weakened walls will tend to rupture. The bronchioles will also become scarred and distorted, becoming kinked on expiration thus causing air-trapping. These mechanisms lead to the development of secondary emphysema.

More rarely, emphysema develops as a primary condition without any previous history of chest disease. Sputum production is unusual in these cases unless there is superimposed infection. The alveolar walls disintegrate over a relatively short period, and the patient will die due to respiratory insufficiency.

In primary emphysema, or when secondary emphysema is predominant, the radiograph will show a low flat diaphragm, a large retrosternal translucent area and bullae may be visible. There will be a narrow vertical heart shadow.

Aims of treatment

1 To remove secretions.
2 To assist relaxation and gain control of breathing.
3 To mobilise the thorax and co-ordinate respiratory movement.
4 To increase the patient's exercise tolerance.

1 Removal of secretions

All patients with chronic bronchitis should carry out regular postural drainage during the productive phases of their disease. (See postural drainage at home, p. 11.) In the absence of infection, the secretions are mucoid. Mucoid secretions are often small in volume and may be removed rapidly, although this may require considerable effort on the part of the patient. Purulent secretions, associated with infection, tend to be larger in volume, and although the patient will be able to expectorate more easily, the treatment will be more prolonged.

In patients with primary emphysema, secretions are usually absent. During an infection sputum may be present and postural drainage is indicated. Emphysema is more commonly 'secondary' and associated with chronic bronchitis, and the removal of secretions is of prime importance. In some patients where emphysema is predominant, tipping may aggravate dyspnoea and postural drainage may need to be modified (p. 11).

Shaking should not be over-vigorous if the patient has been on high maintenance doses of cortico-steroids as there is a tendency to osteoporosis, and rib or vertebral fractures may result.

If the patient is unable to clear his chest adequately, it may be helpful to provide increased ventilation and humidification by means of intermittent positive pressure breathing (IPPB). This in conjunction with postural drainage, will facilitate expectoration (p. 71). There is often an element of bronchospasm present in association with these diseases. If reversible bronchospasm is present, IPPB with a bronchodilator may be given prior to postural drainage (p. 74).

2 Relaxation and control of breathing

During an attack of dyspnoea, the patient

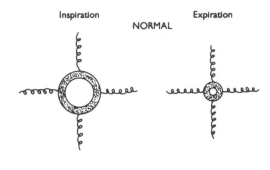

Inspiration   Expiration
NORMAL

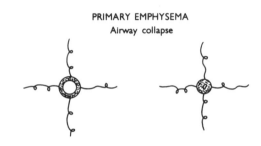

PRIMARY EMPHYSEMA
Airway collapse

Fig. 28. *Airway collapse. By courtesy of Professor Lynne Reid.*

with bronchitis and/or emphysema tends to hold his chest in a position of inspiration. There is over-activity of the accessory muscles, and diaphragmatic movement is inhibited.

The pattern of breathing developed by an emphysematous patient is a short uncontrolled inspiration, using the accessory muscles, followed by a prolonged and often forced expiration. This forced expiration produces a rise in intrathoracic pressure which may cause closure of the airways that are either damaged, or no longer have the support of normal elastic lung tissue (fig. 28). This uncontrolled pattern of breathing is an exhausting and uneconomical method of ventilation, which the physiotherapist should attempt to reverse.

Some emphysematous patients spontaneously develop a technique of 'pursed-lip' breathing. Such patients breathe out through the mouth with the lips held together loosely in a pursed position. By increasing the pressure in the pharynx and upper airways, the damaged collapsible airways are kept patent a little longer, and probably the patient feels relief from the resultant slightly increased tidal volume and slower respiratory rate. This method of breathing should not be discouraged, provided that it is carried out correctly in a relaxed manner. If one attempts to teach this form of breathing to a patient who has not developed it spontaneously, there is a great danger of expiration becoming forced, thus defeating the purpose of the technique. Unless this pattern is already established, it should be omitted from the treatment programme.

All patients with obstructive airways disease are taught to breathe with an active inspiratory phase using the diaphragm, and a passive relaxed expiratory phase. If the

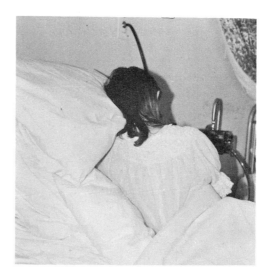

Fig. 30. *High side-lying (posterior aspect).*

patient can control his breathing, it can be of great benefit during attacks of dyspnoea. He is instructed to adopt a relaxed position, as shown in figs. 29 to 34. These positions are all designed to combine the maximum relaxation of the upper chest, with freedom of movement of the lower chest. At this stage the rate of breathing is not important but control of the upper chest is essential. The patient should be encouraged to breathe gently with the lower chest without prolonging expiration, as described on page 5, until he begins to breathe in a more co-ordinated manner. Once this has been achieved, an effort should be made to slow down his respiratory rate and increase the depth of respiration. The patient may prefer to breathe with his mouth open during an attack of dyspnoea. The positions can be adapted to different situations in everyday life.

HIGH SIDE-LYING (figs. 29 and 30)

The patient lies on one side, slightly rolled

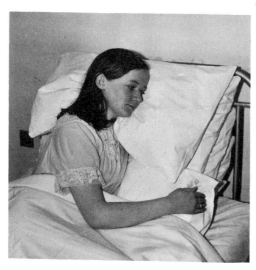

Fig. 29. *High side-lying.*

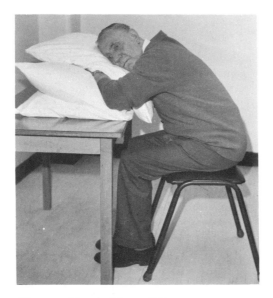

Fig. 31. *Forward lean sitting.*

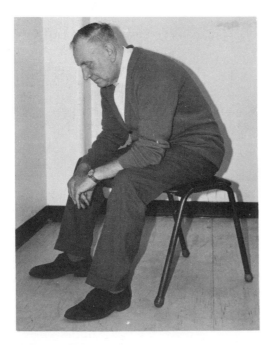

Fig. 32. *Relaxed sitting.*

forward, with a slope of three or four pillows to raise the shoulders, and an extra pillow placed to fill the gap between the waist and axilla to prevent him sliding down the bed and to maintain a straight thoracic spine. The knees are slightly bent and the top leg placed in front of the lower one. This position is helpful for patients in acute respiratory distress, or at night for those suffering from orthopnoea.

FORWARD LEAN SITTING (fig. 31)

Certain patients who prefer not to stay in bed find this position comfortable. Two or three pillows are placed on a table and the patient can relax with the upper chest and head resting against them. Care should be taken that the patient maintains a straight thoracic and lumbar spine as otherwise this would tend to inhibit diaphragmatic movement.

RELAXED SITTING (fig. 32)

This is an extremely useful position and can be taken up unobtrusively in public places. Many patients are inclined to grip their knees and raise their shoulders when in distress, but if they can sit leaning forward with the forearms resting on the thighs, and the wrists relaxed, they will recover more quickly. Care must be taken to ensure that the lumbar spine is not flexed, as this could impede free forward movement of the abdominal wall.

FORWARD LEAN STANDING (fig. 33)

If they are unable to sit down, distressed patients are inclined to grasp the nearest available object and hold themselves in a tense position; for instance they hold on to

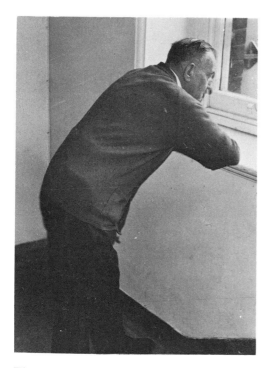

Fig. 33. *Forward lean standing.*

the banisters after climbing a flight of stairs
They should be encouraged to lean forward
as shown in the illustration.

RELAXED STANDING (fig. 34)

The distressed patient may also help himself
by leaning back against the wall or an upright support. The feet should be approximately twelve inches from the wall, the
shoulders relaxed and arms hanging loosely
by the sides.

CONTROL OF BREATHING
DURING EXERCISE

When the patient is able to control his
breathing in these relaxed positions he
should practise while sitting and standing

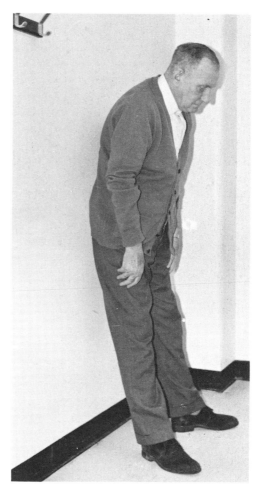

Fig. 34. *Relaxed standing.*

upright without support. Progression can
then be made to control of breathing while
walking on the level, on stairs, and on hills.
Many patients tend to hold their breath
during exercise. Breathing in rhythm with
their steps can be helpful; for example,
breathing out for two steps and in for one
step, or out for three steps and in for two
steps. A breathing pattern must be worked
out for each individual patient.

Some patients tend to become distressed

25

when bending forward (e.g. to tie shoe laces). Many of them breathe in before bending down, and thus experience discomfort due to the upward pressure of the abdominal contents against the flattened diaphragm. This discomfort is alleviated to a certain extent if breathing out is encouraged whilst bending down; breathing in takes place during the return to an upright position.

Although pulmonary function tests do not show any significant improvement in patients who have been taught controlled breathing, they appear to derive benefit from the fact that they are breathing in a more economical manner. By eliminating superfluous muscular activity during respiration, the work of breathing is reduced.

3 Mobilisation of the thorax and co-ordination of respiratory movement

Treatment is not progressed until the patient has mastered breathing control and relaxation of the upper chest, whether during attacks of dyspnoea, or during normal breathing.

Localised basal expansion (p. 6) is then started. This is taught unilaterally and can be progressed to belt exercises. Basal expansion is helpful in loosening secretions during postural drainage. By improving the mobility of the lower thoracic cage together with control of the upper chest, the patient should achieve a more normal co-ordinated pattern of breathing.

In patients with emphysema, the domes of the diaphragm are flattened or even inverted. This abnormal position of the diaphragm can cause rib retraction on inspiration, but with perseverance a little lateral basal movement may eventually be achieved.

4 Increase of exercise tolerance

At one time it was common practice in physiotherapy departments to hold breathing classes for groups of patients; but it is now generally accepted that adults benefit more from individual treatment.

The aim of physiotherapy for severely disabled patients is to increase their exercise tolerance to enable them to carry out useful daily activities. Patients should be encouraged to be as mobile and active as possible. Their exercise tolerance may be increased by improving control of breathing, while gradually increasing the distances walked, both on the level and on slopes and stairs.

A few patients are so handicapped that they may need portable oxygen therapy, and in some cases the assistance of a high walking-frame to enable them to get about (fig. 35).

There is evidence that the improvement in the patient's exercise tolerance with a programme of graduated activities is due to reduced oxygen consumption during exercise although the precise mechanisms by which this occurs are as yet unclear.

A number of research papers have been written on the effects of exercise (bicycle, treadmill and stairs) whilst the patient is using portable oxygen. The consensus of opinion would seem to be that the reduced dyspnoea, and increase in speed and distance walked, is probably related to the opening up of the pulmonary capillary bed (due to reduced pulmonary vascular resistance) and improved oxygen uptake. It is our experience that the use of a bicycle and treadmill as a means of treatment are not particularly advantageous in improving the exercise tolerance in the severely disabled patient,

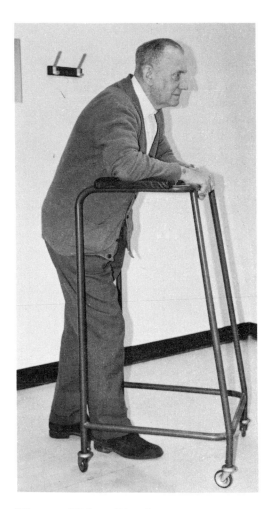

Fig. 35. *High walking frame.*

but that gradually increasing the activities of daily living is more functionally beneficial.

Home instruction

It is essential that all patients with chronic obstructive airways disease carry out physiotherapy at home. Prolonged out-patient treatment is usually unnecessary if careful instructions have been given.

ACUTE EXACERBATIONS OF CHRONIC BRONCHITIS

If a patient with chronic bronchitis develops an acute infection, his condition may deteriorate rapidly. Excess bronchial secretion is produced, and although some is expectorated, a considerable quantity remains in the bronchial tree, so contributing to airways obstruction. Swelling of the bronchial mucosa due to the infection will decrease the lumen of the air passages and further contribute to obstruction. This obstruction to ventilation results in inadequate gas exchange in the periphery of the lung: the Po_2 (oxygen tension) of the arterial blood falls, while the Pco_2 (carbon dioxide tension) of the arterial blood rises. As a result, the patient becomes drowsy and confused, and his breathing becomes erratic, shallow and inefficient.

At this stage, vigorous physiotherapy is essential. The usual methods of postural drainage, shaking, etc., may not be effective because the patient may be unable to co-operate with efficient breathing and coughing. IPPB can be of great value here, and may obviate the need for intubation (p. 71 for techniques with IPPB). Assisted ventilation with vigorous chest shaking, and postural drainage where possible, has the effect of aerating the lungs more efficiently and loosening secretions. The patient often begins to cough spontaneously and becomes more alert. During the early, acute stage of the exacerbation, it may be necessary to repeat the treatment at hourly intervals.

COR PULMONALE

In 1961 the World Health Organization defined cor pulmonale as follows: 'Hypertrophy of the right ventricle resulting from diseases affecting the function and/or structure of the lung, except when these pulmonary alterations are the result of diseases that primarily affect the left side of the heart or of congenital heart disease.'

Cor pulmonale most commonly occurs in association with long-standing pulmonary disease such as chronic bronchitis or bronchiectasis. It is also seen in patients with kypho-scoliosis. It rarely occurs in primary emphysema.

A respiratory infection superimposed on one of these conditions frequently precipitates cor pulmonale. The respiratory infection causes carbon dioxide retention and hypoxia, and these together cause constriction of the pulmonary arterioles so producing pulmonary hypertension. Many pulmonary blood vessels are obliterated by disease of lung tissue, thus making the passage of blood through the pulmonary circulation even more difficult. A radiograph of the chest will show cardiac enlargement and dilatation of the main pulmonary arteries. In the later stages of cor pulmonale, right ventricular failure develops due to the enormous work load and continuing hypoxia.

Energetic physiotherapy, as described for an acute exacerbation of chronic bronchitis, is required to clear excess secretions and to improve alveolar ventilation. Other treatment includes oxygen therapy, antibiotics and diuretics. It must be understood that the right-sided heart failure in cor pulmonale will not be relieved until the chest condition has been treated. Physiotherapy, therefore, is of prime importance.

ASTHMA

Asthma refers to the condition of patients with widespread narrowing of the bronchial airways, which changes in its severity over short periods of time either spontaneously or under treatment, and is not due to cardiovascular disease.

Persistent and severe asthma is described as status asthmaticus; in this condition the bronchi may have become plugged with tenacious exudate and casts. On admission to hospital, the patient will be extremely short of breath and frequently exhausted. Drug and oxygen therapy will be instituted immediately, and physiotherapy will usually be requested soon after admission. Patients with a widely varying degree of asthma ranging from those in status asthmaticus to those who are almost symptom free will be treated by physiotherapy.

Aims of physiotherapy

1 To relieve bronchospasm.
2 To assist relaxation and gain control of breathing.
3 To aid removal of secretions.
4 To co-ordinate respiratory movement.

1 Relief of bronchospasm

This is the most important aspect of the treatment as it will be impossible to mobilise the secretions until the bronchospasm has been relieved. It is important for the physiotherapist to remember that coughing and postural drainage may aggravate bronchospasm.

Administration of a bronchodilator by means of IPPB is often very effective (p. 74). The patient should be in a comfortable position, either sitting upright, well supported by pillows, or in a high side-lying position. IPPB with the prescribed bronchodilator should be given and the patient encouraged to relax and breathe with his diaphragm.

2 Relaxation and control of breathing

Relaxation and control of breathing are important in both severe and mild asthma. The patient should be shown the relaxed positions described on p. 23–25, and encouraged to breathe gently with his diaphragm at his own rate during attacks of dyspnoea. He should only be encouraged to slow down his rate of respiration once he has gained control.

3 Removal of secretions

Great care must be taken not to aggravate bronchospasm when assisting with removal of secretions; if a patient is unable to expectorate, the physiotherapist should not persist with this treatment but wait until further bronchodilatation has taken place.

Once the secretions have started to liquefy, the physiotherapist should give gentle chest vibrations on expiration, with the patient in the high side-lying position. This treatment should be given ten to fifteen minutes after administration of a bronchodilator. At this stage, many patients start to expectorate thick, tenacious sputum which frequently contains casts. As the patient's condition improves, vibrations can be given in the side-lying position, and when he can tolerate it, the bed may be tipped.

4 Co-ordination of respiratory movement

Localised basal expansion exercises should be started when there is improvement in the patient's condition. The patient should be made aware of his pattern of breathing, and should be encouraged to relax the upper chest and eliminate the action of the accessory muscles. It is often helpful to practise in front of a mirror, as many patients are unaware of their faulty pattern of breathing.

Exercise for asthmatics

It is a well-known fact that exercise may induce bronchoconstriction in asthmatic patients. Research is being carried out into the effects of exercise in these patients, and it has been found that there are significantly smaller falls in FEV$_1$ after swimming than after running and bicycling. The aetiology of increased airways resistance after exercise is still unexplained, but recent studies indicate that swimming should be recommended in preference to bicycling or running.

Children with asthma often have poor posture and frequently do not participate in physical training in school. Many of them enjoy class work and often benefit from being treated in groups. It is a wise precaution to measure the FEV$_1$ or peak flow rate of these patients whenever they attend for treatment. If the readings are low, thus indicating an increase in airways obstruction, they should not join in the class, and treatment should consist of administration of the prescribed bronchodilator followed by removal of secretions, relaxation and breathing control. During classes for asthmatic patients, the more vigorous exercises should not last longer than three minutes at a time, and should be interspersed with relaxation and breathing control.

With the prophylactic use of disodium chromoglycate (Intal), many children with asthma are able to lead relatively normal lives, and once instruction has been given in breathing control and postural drainage, it should not be necessary to continue to attend the physiotherapy department. Swimming should be encouraged, as it is an ideal form of exercise for asthmatics.

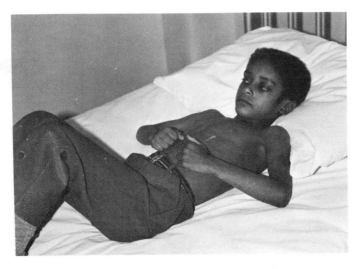

Fig. 36. *Diaphragmatic breathing.*

BRONCHITIS AND ASTHMA IN CHILDREN

Recurrent 'chestiness' in children is a very common condition. Some children even react to mild upper respiratory tract infections by coughing and wheezing, and sometimes it may be difficult to make a clear distinction between bronchitis and asthma.

Babies and children respond well to postural drainage if they have excessive secretions, and from the age of three upwards it is possible to teach breathing exercises. The habit of mouth breathing should be discouraged. The principles of treatment are the same as for an adult, with modification of some positions (figs. 36–39).

Instructions should be given to parents in supervision of exercises at home, and in assistance to the child during an asthma attack. Breathing exercises should be practised daily for at least ten minutes, and it is often necessary to carry out postural drainage.

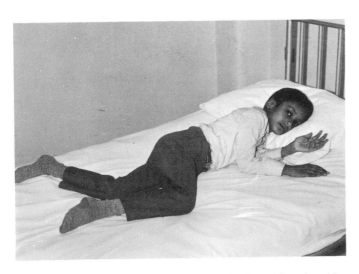

Fig. 37. *Diaphragmatic breathing in side-lying.*

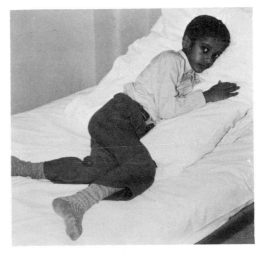

Fig. 38. *High side-lying.*

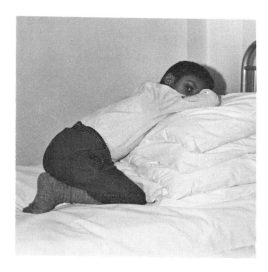

Fig. 39. *Kneeling position for breathlessness.*

PULMONARY INFECTIONS AND ASSOCIATED DISEASES

PNEUMONIA

Acute lobar pneumonia is not often seen in hospital since it responds quickly to antibiotic therapy if this is started in the early stages. However, from time to time cases are admitted, and if physiotherapy is requested the treatment must not be confused with that appropriate for the more common bronchopneumonia.

Acute lobar pneumonia is characterised by fever, malaise and toxaemia. Pulmonary consolidation is present in one or more lobes, and it is frequently due to infection by the pneumococcus. In the early stages of the disease the patient suffers from pleuritic pain, dyspnoea and a painful cough. Pleuritic pain is an acute localised chest pain, worse on coughing or deep breathing, and is due to inflammation of the pleura overlying the consolidated lobe. The cough is usually unproductive, but there may be scanty tenacious mucoid sputum, or it may be blood-stained and 'rusty' in colour. An area of consolidation will be apparent on radiography. During this stage localised breathing exercises are encouraged; chest shaking and percussion are not only painful but of no benefit to the patient.

In the next stages of the disease, the pulmonary consolidation starts to resolve, and as the pleuritic pain diminishes coughing becomes less painful and usually productive of mucopurulent sputum. At this stage appropriate postural drainage is instituted and assistance given to clear secretions.

Bronchopneumonia, in contrast to lobar pneumonia, is patchy in distribution and is associated primarily with bronchial inflammatory change. It is seen more frequently than lobar pneumonia, and commonly in post-operative patients and in chronic bronchitics, and especially when these two situations co-exist. Physiotherapy is an essential part of the treatment regime and is instituted immediately. Purulent or mucopurulent sputum is present in considerable quantities causing obstruction of the airways. As there is no consolidation or pleural inflammation causing pleuritic pain, there is no contra-indication to early physiotherapy. This consists of breathing exercises combined with postural drainage, percussion and chest shaking to assist the removal of secretions. If these measures are not effective, IPPB is used to assist ventilation and clearing of secretions (p. 71).

LUNG ABSCESS

Postural drainage is started as soon as the diagnosis of lung abscess is made. The abscess sometimes causes distortion of the bronchi, and therefore postural drainage positions may have to be modified in order to obtain effective drainage.

It is unwise to give breathing exercises until the radiograph shows some diminution in the size of the abscess. An increase in size is an indication of air trapping and expansion exercises would aggravate the situation. Once the abscess begins to decrease in size, expansion exercises are given to assist the postural drainage in removal of secretions.

BRONCHIECTASIS

Bronchiectasis is characterised by dilatation of the bronchi associated with obstruction and infection. It may be caused by pulmonary collapse associated with pneumonia, or more rarely by obstruction of a bronchus as in primary tuberculosis (p. 34). The diagnosis will be confirmed by a bronchogram.

Most patients have a productive cough with purulent sputum and suffer from repeated chest infections. Haemoptysis may occur in varying degrees, and in some patients it may be their only symptom; this is known as 'dry' bronchiectasis.

Destruction of the cilia which are responsible for clearing the bronchi will have occurred as a result of the disease. Postural drainage is therefore essential for patients with a productive cough. Even if the cilia survive, they may beat ineffectively due to the excessive secretions. These patients will have to continue postural drainage for the rest of their lives and therefore instruction in home management is vital.

Postural drainage is unnecessary for patients with 'dry' bronchiectasis; it may even aggravate the tendency to haemoptysis. If a mild haemoptysis occurs in productive patients, postural drainage may be continued, but it is probably wiser to omit percussion for the next twenty-four hours. If severe haemoptysis occurs, physiotherapy should be discontinued temporarily until the bleeding has been controlled.

If the disease is sufficiently localised, some patients may undergo surgery for removal of the affected lobe or lobes (p. 49).

CYSTIC FIBROSIS

Cystic fibrosis is a genetically determined disorder which has become increasingly recognised since it was first described in 1938. In this condition the exocrine glands are abnormal and the patients have an unusually high concentration of sodium in the sweat; abnormal pancreatic function and recurrent lung infections occur either together or separately. The abnormal pancreatic function results in malabsorption and steatorrhoea, and the recurrent lung infections result in generalised suppurative bronchiectasis and the formation of multiple lung abscesses. The survival of these patients depends on the control of pulmonary infection and prevention of permanent lung damage. At one time it was unusual for these patients to survive over the age of 14, but with improved diagnosis and treatment many patients are now surviving to over the age of 30.

The introduction of postural drainage even before chest symptoms and signs have appeared is recommended, as present evidence suggests that this may delay the onset of chest complications and improve the overall prognosis. It should be remembered that radiological changes may be present without any detectable clinical change.

Treatment of the pulmonary complications consists of appropriate antibiotics and physiotherapy. Although antibiotic requirements may vary from time to time, physiotherapy must be a constant feature of the management even when the patient is apparently 'well'. During an exacerbation it is absolutely imperative that intensive physiotherapy is carried out. Even though the patient may attend a specialist hospital at intervals for follow up, the local hospital should be prepared to offer facilities for physiotherapy if the patient and his relatives are unable to manage at home on these occasions.

The frequency and duration of *postural drainage* must be carefully assessed for each individual and the appropriate positions taught for the affected areas of the lungs. During an exacerbation the patient may need to spend as long as thirty minutes draining each area, and it is often necessary to carry out treatment six times a day. In hospital the nursing staff should be asked, whenever possible, to position the patient early in the morning and late in the evening.

Often the lower lobes and mid-zones are all affected, and in order to give the patient some respite, the physiotherapist may have to be satisfied with treating both lower lobes at one session and the mid-zones at the next session.

The home programme must be worked out for each individual. Relatives should be instructed in the postural drainage positions appropriate for the patient, and be shown how to perform clapping and shaking correctly. It is essential that they realise the vital importance of regular treatment and encourage the patient to continue this conscientiously. Postural drainage should not be given immediately following a meal. Infants should be treated just before their feeds. Patients who produce sputum only occasionally, should carry out postural drainage once or twice a day. Early in the morning, and/or before going to bed in the evening, are usually the most suitable times. If no specific area is apparently causing trouble, the positions for draining the lateral and posterior segments of both lower lobes are probably the most suitable to teach. If the patient has a cold, treatment must be performed more frequently until the excessive production of sputum has subsided.

A physiotherapist should see the patient at regular intervals (for instance when he attends the doctor's follow-up clinic), in order to assess the chest condition, suggest any alterations in home treatment and discuss any problems that have arisen.

Difficulties are often encountered in the treatment of adolescents who become resentful of their condition and authority in general; they may rebel against any form of treatment given by their parents or doctors. In this situation it is often better for the physiotherapist to see the patient without his parents and to try to persuade him of the importance of regular drainage, and to offer facilities for out-patient physiotherapy when feasible. After the patient has left school there may be a problem of fitting in the treatment around his hours of work, but a solution must be worked out.

Breathing exercises should be an integral part of the postural drainage treatment; emphasis must be on relaxed expiration. Diaphragmatic breathing and basal expansion exercises should be practised regularly as there is a tendency to develop an over-inflated upper chest.

Participation in physical education should be encouraged; *general activities* such as swimming and running are also beneficial.

Some authorities feel that the regular use of *mist tents* in the management of these patients is essential, others feel that it is only necessary during an acute infective exacerbation. Patients with thick tenacious secretions often find it easier to expectorate after a period in a mist tent.

In this country many patients use a small *inhalation* apparatus providing mist therapy via a mouthpiece or mask. The use of this before or during postural drainage helps to moisten the air passages and ease the removal of secretions. If bronchospasm is present, it may be relieved by inhalation of a bronchodilator before treatment. If antibiotics are given via the nebuliser, this should be done after postural drainage. IPPB should be used with caution when treating cystic fibrosis because of the possibility of causing a pneumothorax.

PULMONARY TUBERCULOSIS

Pulmonary tuberculosis has become less common since the improvement of public health standards and treatment by effective chemotherapy. Physiotherapy is rarely requested for this condition, but it is sometimes necessary to treat associated complications.

The first infection with the tubercle bacillus is known as *primary tuberculosis*. A small pneumonic lesion may occur in any part of the lung and the nearest lymph glands become enlarged. The lesion usually heals by fibrosis and calcification and subsequently causes no problem; occasionally it spreads through the lobe and may then cavitate. If pleural effusion occurs, localised expansion exercises are required (p. 6).

In infants and young children, the enlarged hilar lymph nodes may compress a bronchus and cause segmental collapse. Prolonged compression may lead to permanent bronchiectasis as in the '*middle lobe syndrome*'. Another cause of segmental collapse may be discharge of caseous material from the affected lymph gland into the bronchus. Physiotherapy may be requested to attempt re-expansion of a collapsed middle lobe. The result may be disappointing but it is worth persevering with breathing exercises, postural drainage and vibrations as re-expansion sometimes occurs.

Post-primary tuberculosis is a re-infection after the primary lesion. The infection usually occurs in the upper lobes or apical segments of the lower lobes. A small area of tuberculous bronchopneumonia appears at first, and this spreads by direct infection to neighbouring lung tissue. Caseation follows, and the necrotic centre of the lesion is discharged into a bronchus, leaving a cavity. The patient coughs up infective sputum, some of which may be inhaled into other areas of lung, producing new tuberculous lesions. Haemoptysis occurs if there is erosion of blood vessels.

Peripheral lesions may cause pleurisy leading to *tuberculous effusion* or *empyema*. In these cases physiotherapy is important to prevent chest deformity and loss of respiratory function by pleural thickening (p. 37). There is no risk of physiotherapy causing spread of the disease once medical treatment has been established.

In contrast to acute tuberculosis with infiltration and cavitation, a *chronic fibro-caseous* condition may develop. Gross fibrous contraction of the upper lobes with compensatory emphysema of the lower lobes results in dyspnoea and diminished respiratory reserve. Breathing control and assistance with removal of secretions, during periods of superimposed chest infection, may be helpful. IPPB may be contra-indicated if cavitation has taken place.

A *tuberculoma* is a cavity with thick walls containing inspissated material which appears radiologically as a rounded opacity. It may be removed surgically since it is sometimes difficult to differentiate tuberculoma from carcinoma.

Tuberculous bronchiectasis may be a complication of either primary or post-primary tuberculosis. Postural drainage may be given, but percussion will be contra-indicated if there is a large cavity, or haemoptysis is occurring. The physiotherapist should stand behind the patient when he is coughing. Treatment is carried out two or three times daily according to the quantity of sputum.

MISCELLANEOUS PULMONARY DISEASES

OCCUPATIONAL LUNG DISEASE

Several lung diseases are attributable to the inhalation of dusts, fumes or noxious substances. The most common of these 'occupational' lung diseases are *coalminers' pneumoconiosis* and *silicosis*.

Fibrotic nodules develop throughout the lungs around the particles of inhaled dust, and these progress to large areas of fibrosis. The diseases may be complicated by chronic bronchitis and emphysematous changes. Symptoms include progressive dyspnoea on exertion, accompanied by cough which may be productive of mucoid sputum and recurrent exacerbations of bronchitis.

The most important aspect of management of these diseases is prevention by adequate precautions in industry, and regular chest radiography for employees exposed to risk.

The aims of physiotherapy are similar to those for chronic bronchitis and emphysema: assistance with removal of secretions by postural drainage, and possibly IPPB (p. 71), and instruction in breathing with the minimum amount of effort.

DIFFUSE FIBROSING ALVEOLITIS

This condition is characterised by a diffuse inflammatory process in the lung beyond the terminal bronchiole, resulting in thickening and fibrosis of the alveolar walls. This may occur rapidly in the subacute form known as the Hamman–Rich syndrome, and it may be fatal within six months. More commonly the disease progresses in the chronic form over a few years.

The characteristic symptom is progressive and unremitting dyspnoea. The main defect found on respiratory function tests is restriction with poor gas exchange measurements. Radiographs show fine, diffuse mottling.

Steroids may limit the fibrosis and relieve dyspnoea in some patients. Physiotherapy is purely palliative. Instruction in breathing control may give some relief. If superimposed infections occur, IPPB and chest vibrations may assist removal of secretions.

ASPERGILLOSIS

This is the most common fungal disease affecting the respiratory system in Great Britain. The spores of the fungus are frequently found in the atmosphere and some people develop an obstructive airways disorder known as *allergic bronchial aspergillosis*. The symptoms include inflammation and oedema of the bronchi and bronchioli which cause wheezing and possible collapse of a segment or lobe due to obstruction. The sputum may contain bronchial casts, often brown in colour, from which *Aspergillus fumigatus* can be cultured.

Treatment is similar to that for asthma, but whereas shaking with postural drainage may not be indicated for an asthmatic, it is always necessary in the treatment of aspergillosis. Postural drainage may take longer than usual if the patient has bronchial casts, but great relief is felt once they are expectorated. IPPB with a bronchodilator preceding postural drainage is useful to relieve bronchospasm (p. 74).

The *Aspergillus fumigatus* may infect cysts or cavities which have resulted from such diseases as tuberculosis, pulmonary infarction or lung abscess. An *aspergilloma* is a solid ball of fungus (mycetoma) which fills the cavity. Radiography will demonstrate a crescent of air above the opacity, which can be shown to alter position with changes of posture.

Some patients have recurrent haemoptysis or repeated infections with thick purulent sputum. Others may be asymptomatic. An aspergilloma is often left untreated, but if haemoptyses are severe, resection may be necessary. There is a risk of spreading the fungal infection and surgery is therefore rarely undertaken.

PULMONARY TUMOURS

Carcinoma of the bronchus is the most common tumour of the lung. The majority of these tumours arise centrally in the larger bronchi and are visible through a bronchoscope. A few develop peripherally. Histologically 56% are found to be squamous cell carcinoma, 37% are anaplastic (oat cell carcinoma), 6% adenocarcinoma and 1% alveolar cell carcinoma.

The first symptoms are often a dry cough and pain, but as the growth increases in size it causes progressive bronchial obstruction and production of mucopurulent sputum, leading eventually to collapse of the lung segment. Haemoptysis may result from ulceration of blood vessels and a persistent wheeze becomes apparent due to obstruction of the bronchus. Complications such as unresolved pneumonia, lung abcess or pleural effusion are not uncommon.

Surgery by lobectomy or pneumonectomy is often the treatment of choice (p. 39), but if the growth is too extensive, or too rapidly progressive (anaplastic), or the respiratory reserve is inadequate, other methods are employed.

Radiotherapy may be used to produce a remission in patients unsuitable for resection, or to relieve symptoms such as obstruction of the superior vena cava. If there is infection beyond the bronchial obstruction the patient will start to expectorate purulent sputum once the tumour reduces in size. Physiotherapy by means of postural drainage and gentle vibrations can help the removal of secretions. Percussion and vigorous shaking are contraindicated in view of possible haemoptysis or the presence of metastases in the spine or ribs.

As a result of radiotherapy, pulmonary fibrosis may develop causing dyspnoea. Instruction in breathing control, particularly when walking, is beneficial.

Physiotherapy may be requested for patients in the terminal stage of the disease to assist with removal of secretions. Postural drainage (or a modified form) with gentle vibrations may be helpful if a patient is distressed and having difficulty in clearing the airways. If the patient is unable to cough and expectorate, is alert and in extreme distress, naso-tracheal suction may on rare occasions be used. However, it is unjustified during the terminal stage if the patient is in a state of coma.

Adenoma and *hamartoma* are benign tumours of the lung treated by surgical removal.

PULMONARY EMBOLISM

A pulmonary embolus most commonly arises from a deep vein thrombosis in the leg or pelvis. A distinction must be drawn between massive pulmonary embolism where more than 50% of the major pulmonary artery branches are obstructed, and pulmonary infarct caused by several small emboli.

Massive pulmonary embolism

A large embolus may cause sudden death. If the embolism is not immediately fatal the patient becomes suddenly shocked, dyspnoeic and complains of central chest pain. Pulmonary angiography may be used to confirm the diagnosis. Treatment may be either by intravenous anti-coagulants or emergency embolectomy. Surgery is carried out on cardiopulmonary bypass (p. 63).

Pulmonary infarction

Small emboli cause a pulmonary infarct. Diagnosis is often difficult, and therefore this serious respiratory lesion is sometimes overlooked. When the infarct extends to the lung surface, the pleura becomes involved causing acute pleuritic pain and often effusion. Haemoptysis only occurs in about 50% of cases, and the source of the embolus is not always clinically detectable. Repeated small emboli may eventually lead to obstruction of the pulmonary vascular bed, and cause pulmonary hypertension and right ventricular failure.

Treatment of pulmonary infarction consists of anti-coagulants, oxygen, bed rest, and analgesia to relieve the pleuritic pain.

Physiotherapy is primarily prophylactic and all patients at risk are given active leg exercises and breathing exercises to assist the venous return. Patients are encouraged to carry out foot and leg exercises at frequent intervals until they are ambulant.

If a pulmonary infarct occurs, physiotherapy is discontinued until anti-coagulant therapy is established. Breathing exercises are given to encourage movement of the affected area since chest movement is limited by the pleuritic pain. Postural drainage may assist expectoration of old blood and clot. Leg exercises are continued until the patient is ambulant.

DISEASES OF THE PLEURAL CAVITY

PLEURAL EFFUSION

Breathing exercises are important following a pleural effusion, in order to maintain mobility of the thoracic cage before adhesions form and the pleura becomes thickened. The types of pleural effusions most commonly seen by the physiotherapist are those found in association with pneumonia, tuberculosis and trauma, and those following thoracic surgery. Pleural effusion may also be associated with cardiac failure, nephritis or intrathoracic neoplasms; these conditions do not benefit from physiotherapy.

If there is a large effusion causing dyspnoea, breathing exercises are not usually effective until the fluid has been aspirated. Expansion exercises are given to all areas of the affected side of the chest, including the apical area where there is often some flattening. Belt exercises are useful in this condition. If there is gross deformity of the chest wall, the patient is positioned lying on the unaffected side with two or three pillows under the thorax in order to open out the rib cage of the affected side. Breathing exercises are done intermittently while in this position. It may be necessary to adopt the position for twenty to thirty minutes several times a day.

EMPYEMA

Empyema, a collection of pus in the pleural cavity, is now rarely seen. It may be associated with bronchopleural fistula following pulmonary surgery. Empyema may be treated surgically by decortication (p. 53) or rib resection with insertion of a drainage tube, or medically. If patients are treated medically, by chemotherapy and possibly aspiration, localised expansion exercises are part of the general treatment regime. Empyema results in thickening of the pleura and restriction of lung movement. Early physiotherapy is essential so that maximum re-expansion of lung tissue and minimum permanent restriction result. Breathing exercises for all areas of the chest are necessary to prevent deformities, as with pleural effusion.

SPONTANEOUS PNEUMOTHORAX

A collection of air in the pleural cavity resulting from some pathological process, is known as spontaneous pneumothorax. When the pneumothorax is small the lung often re-expands within a few days. Treatment consists of rest alone; physiotherapy is usually unnecessary. If the lung fails to re-expand, or collapses further, air must be withdrawn from the pleural cavity; an intercostal tube is inserted for a few days and the air in the pleural space withdrawn. Following the insertion of a tube, breathing exercises may be given to assist re-expansion of the lung; particular attention should be given to expansion of the apical region. The physiotherapist should ensure that the patient carries out a full range of movements in the shoulder joint.

In some cases the spontaneous pneumothorax recurs with consequent chest pain, dyspnoea and interference with day-to-day activities. Moreover, if any other lung disease is present such as emphysema, a recurrent pneumothorax may result in severe disability. For this reason the pleural cavity is often obliterated medically with talc or irritant oils (pleurodesis), or surgically by pleurectomy (p. 52).

5 Surgical conditions

PULMONARY SURGERY

This section deals primarily with physiotherapy associated with surgery of the lungs and pleura, but also includes oesophageal and diaphragmatic surgery and correction of chest deformities. The general principles of physiotherapy are considered first, and then details for the individual operations follow (p. 49).

Physiotherapy has an important part to play in the care of patients following pulmonary surgery, and one of the aids to a quick recovery is adequate pre-operative training. The principles of pre-operative treatment are the same for all patients undergoing chest surgery, but obviously vary in detail according to the individual's condition and the operation performed. Treatment should start as early as possible, preferably at least five days before surgery. Some patients however, may be admitted only a day or two before operation, and in these instances treatment would probably be required at least twice a day.

Before starting pre-operative treatment, the physiotherapist should examine the patient's medical history and chest radiographs, and any other relevant investigations such as respiratory function tests. It is important at this stage that the physiotherapist evaluates the patient's normal breathing pattern and his thoracic mobility. These observations should be recorded, as they will be of value in the post-operative phase.

Aims of physiotherapy following pulmonary surgery

1 To preserve adequate ventilation.
2 To assist removal of excessive secretions from the airways and thereby prevent post-operative pulmonary collapse.
3 To maintain or regain full expansion of the remaining lung tissue.
4 To assist the circulation of the legs, and thereby help prevent post-operative venous thrombosis.
5 To maintain mobility of the shoulders, shoulder girdle, spine and chest.
6 To prevent postural defects.
7 To restore exercise tolerance.

PRE-OPERATIVE TRAINING

1 Explanation to the patient

During the pre-operative period, the physiotherapist should gain the patient's confidence in order that he will be prepared to co-operate after his operation, despite discomfort.

It must be explained that to maintain adequate ventilation of the lungs, deep breathing must be performed which will inevitably cause a certain amount of pain. He should be told that although sedation will be given, this does not eliminate pain entirely. He must understand the importance of clearing secretions present in the airways after surgery, in order to prevent post-operative complications. Reassurance must be given that deep breathing, coughing and moving around in bed, will in no way harm the stitches, drainage tubes or operation site.

The patient should also realise the importance of starting his exercises as soon as he recovers consciousness after surgery, and that physiotherapy is of the greatest importance during the first few post-operative days.

2 Removal of secretions

The lungs should be as clear as possible before operation, and any excessive secretions must be removed by appropriate postural drainage. If bronchiectasis is present, postural drainage will probably be necessary at least four times a day.

Cigarette smoking causes bronchoconstriction and excessive secretions, and the patient should be encouraged to stop as soon as possible.

Bronchitis often co-exists with bronchial carcinoma, and some patients may be too dyspnoeic to tolerate the true postural drainage positions for the lung bases; in such instances a modified form should be used (p. 11).

3 Breathing exercises

(a) DIAPHRAGMATIC BREATHING (p. 5).

This exercise assists the loosening of secretions by aerating the lower zones of the lungs. Encouragement should be given to relax the upper chest and shoulder girdle in order to perform the exercise correctly.

(b) UNILATERAL BASAL EXPANSION (p. 6).

A lateral thoracotomy is used for the majority of operations included in this section. For all such operations, with the exception of pneumonectomy, the patient will be required to emphasise lateral basal expansion for the side of the incision, since movement of this side will be inhibited by pain. Unilateral expansion of the unaffected side should also be practised to assist with improving ventilation. Holding full inspiration for one or two seconds, during each breath taken, helps in aeration of the alveoli.

At the present time, most pulmonary surgery is performed for bronchial carcinoma. The surgeon may not always be able to predict the scope of an operation until the chest has been opened. Lobectomy may be possible, or it may be necessary to remove the entire lung. Occasionally the growth is so extensive as to make the case inoperable. It is best to prepare the patient as for a lobectomy, but to warn him that post-operatively he may have to rest the operation side for a few days and concentrate on the other side (in case a pneumonectomy is performed). Reassurance must be given that he will be told exactly what to do when he recovers from the anaesthetic. The physiotherapist is then able to avoid answering awkward questions as to the precise nature of the operation. It is the surgeon, not the physiotherapist, who should tell the patient the details of the operation.

(c) APICAL EXPANSION (p. 7).

This exercise assists re-expansion of remaining lung tissue, helps to prevent the formation of an apical airpocket, and prevents a flattening deformity of the upper chest.

In summary, pre-operatively all patients should be taught: (a) diaphragmatic breathing; (b) unilateral basal expansion for both sides of the chest, with special emphasis on the incision side (except for those *known* to be undergoing pneumonectomy); (c) apical expansion for the operation side (except for pneumonectomy).

4 Effective coughing

Prior to coughing, a type of forced expiration, 'huffing', is helpful to loosen secretions and to initiate coughing in post-operative patients. To 'huff' correctly the patient takes a full inspiration using the diaphragm, and then breathes out sharply, contracting the abdominal muscles firmly. The vocal cords should remain open, and there should be a 'breathy' noise produced as distinct from the sharp explosive noise of a cough.

After two or three efficient 'huffs', the patient should inspire deeply again and give two strong coughs with the mouth slightly open. The abdominal muscles must be contracted during the expiratory coughing phase.

The patient must be aware of the difference between an effective cough and a noise created in the throat. The physiotherapist should also attune herself to the various coughing sounds that patients make, so that she is not misled by a dry coughing noise when secretions might be heard and shifted if the cough were deeper and more effective.

N.B. Forced expiration, 'huffing', should be used with caution in patients suffering from obstructive airways disease (p. 6). If such a patient undergoes thoracic surgery, it should be explained that this exercise may be necessary to help shift secretions for a few days after surgery, but

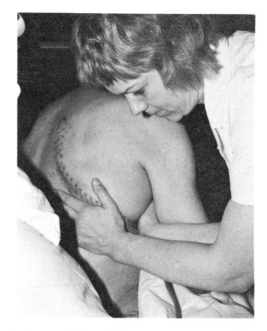

Fig. 40. *Lateral thoracotomy supported by physiotherapist.*

should not be done at any other time as it may increase airways obstruction.

The physiotherapist should show the patient how she will support the chest firmly just below the incision for a lateral thoracotomy (fig. 40), and how he can support himself in order to relieve the discomfort when 'huffing' and coughing after the operation. He should place the arm of the unaffected side across the front of the chest, the hand giving pressure just below the incision and the other elbow giving pressure inwards to the chest wall (fig. 41).

A series of the necessary breathing exercises (in groups of six at a time) should be practised by the patient three or four times a day during the pre-operative period. These should be followed by a few effective 'huffs' and coughs.

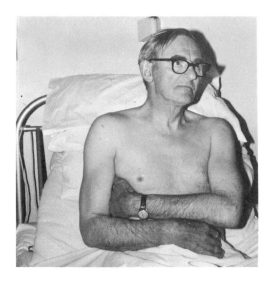

Fig. 41. *Lateral thoracotomy supported by patient.*

5 Foot and leg exercises

All patients should be taught simple foot exercises and knee flexion and extension in order to assist the circulation and help prevent post-operative venous thrombosis. The importance of practising these movements several times during every waking hour until he is able to walk around in the ward, should be stressed to the patient.

6 Posture

The habitual standing posture of the patient should be noted in order that a comparison can be made with posture during the post-operative period.

Nowadays patients are ambulant very soon after surgery and problems of postural deformity rarely arise, but children and young adults sometimes find difficulty in maintaining good posture after lateral thoracotomy. The tendency to side-flex

the trunk towards the incision and to lower the affected shoulder should be pointed out to the patient; and the importance of correcting this tendency and thereby preventing any permanent defect, should be explained (fig. 42).

7 Arm and shoulder girdle movements

Any restriction in shoulder joint movement should be recorded pre-operatively. The prevention of loss of joint range and mobility by early post-operative shoulder girdle and arm exercises should be explained to the patient. Simple shoulder girdle and arm exercises should be briefly practised. Resisted movement with proprioceptive neuromuscular facilitation techniques are helpful in gaining full range with minimal pain; it is worth while practising a few movements with this technique pre-operatively.

8 Moving in bed

It is helpful to show the patient how to

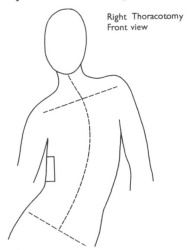

Right Thoracotomy
Front view

Fig. 42. *Postural defects after thoracotomy.*

move himself up the bed taking his weight on his unaffected arm so that he can be mobile without pulling on his drainage tubes and causing pain.

POST-OPERATIVE TREATMENT

Before starting treatment, the physiotherapist should read the operation notes to find out the details of the procedure performed.

Before each treatment the patient should be observed and his record charts studied:

1 Colour, cyanosis.
2 Respiratory rate.
3 Temperature and pulse.
4 Blood pressure.
5 Drainage from pleural drain; bubbling or swing in bottles.
6 Blood gas results.
7 Sputum expectorated; colour and quantity.
8 Chest radiograph.
9 Analgesia; note the time the last dose was given.
10 It is helpful to listen to the breath sounds before and after treatment if familiar with the use of a stethoscope.

DAY OF OPERATION

Post-operative treatment should start after return to the ward, when the patient is sufficiently conscious and co-operative. He should be encouraged to do his breathing exercises and then, while firmly supported, be helped to cough. Often he will cough better at this stage than on the following day as there may be residual analgesia and sedation from the anaesthetic.

FIRST AND SECOND DAYS AFTER OPERATION

Treatment is probably necessary four times during the day. The patient should be sitting up in bed with the spine well supported by pillows, so that there is no kyphosis or scoliosis to inhibit diaphragmatic and chest movement. After about twenty-four hours the patient will normally be allowed to sit out of bed in an armchair for short periods. The exercises can be carried out satisfactorily in this position.

Treatment should consist of:

1 Breathing exercises

(a) Diaphragmatic breathing.
(b) Unilateral basal expansion for both sides of the chest with emphasis on the operation side (except after pneumonectomy).
(c) Apical expansion if appropriate.
It is essential at this stage to obtain full re-expansion of the remaining lung tissue and to prevent retention of excessive secretions that might cause segmental or lobar collapse.

2 Coughing

Effective 'huffing' and coughing, as taught pre-operatively (p. 41), must be encouraged with the chest firmly supported. The patient often finds it easier to cough while sitting forwards in bed away from the pillows. When helping to sit the patient forward, support should be given behind the neck to avoid pulling on the painful arm.

3 Shoulder movements

Shoulder movements should be started the morning after the operation. Resistance given with proprioceptive neuromuscular facilitation techniques is helpful in achieving a good range of movement with minimal pain.

4 Foot and leg exercises

The exercises taught pre-operatively should be practised and the patient should be reminded to do each exercise 5–10 times every hour that he is awake.

5 Postural drainage

If the chest radiograph is satisfactory, the breath sounds adequate on auscultation, and the patient able to breathe deeply and cough effectively, there is probably no need to put him through the unnecessary discomfort of postural drainage.

If there is much sputum and the patient is having difficulty in clearing it, postural drainage will probably be necessary. Some surgeons leave the decision to the physiotherapist, others prefer to be consulted first. The decision usually rests on how well the patient is in other respects.

A patient suffering from bronchiectasis should definitely have postural drainage.

The drainage position most helpful at this stage (except for pneumonectomy, p. 50) is for the lateral basal segment of the affected lung base. The patient is laid flat, turned on to his unaffected side, supported by pillows and the foot of the bed raised. The degree to which the bed is tipped depends on the condition of the patient. It is essential that the shoulder does not rest on the head pillows, and that the arm on the operated side is supported by a pillow. The drainage tubes should be supported by a pillow behind the back.

Analgesia

Analgesics are given at regular intervals during the first 48 hours after surgery in order to reduce pain, but not in such quantities as to produce respiratory depression. If the patient is in much pain and unable to perform the breathing exercises adequately, the physiotherapist should ascertain whether more analgesia can be given and arrange to carry out the treatment when it has taken effect.

Inhalational analgesics such as Entonox or Penthrane may assist effective deep breathing exercises.

Inhalations

A simple steam inhalation before physiotherapy can help in loosening sticky secretions, provided the patient inspires deeply. If bronchospasm is present, a bronchodilator may be necessary before treatment.

The patient may be dehydrated at this early stage, and sometimes a drink helps with coughing and expectoration.

Drainage tubes

After most operations with lateral thoracotomy incisions there will be at least two drainage tubes from the pleural cavity to underwater seal drainage bottles. The basal tube drains fluid, and the apical tube allows air leaking from lung tissue into the pleural space to escape, thereby keeping the lung expanded. The basal tube is normally removed within 24 hours of surgery. The apical drain (or drains) remains until there is no air leak; this is noted by air bubbling through the drainage bottles during coughing. If it is removed too early, a pneumothorax results and another tube may have to be inserted.

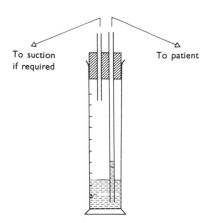

To suction if required

To patient

Fig. 43. *Underwater seal drainage.*

Each tube is connected via an air-tight bung to a bottle partly filled with sterile water so that air cannot enter the pleura. This is known as an underwater seal. The bottle also has an open tube to allow displacement of air. As air comes out of the pleural cavity it bubbles through the water and out of the bottle (fig. 43).

To help keep the remaining lung expanded, the exit tube is usually connected to a suction pump so that a negative pressure is maintained in the bottle. The negative pressure should be increased if a large air leak is present.

If no suction pump is used, there is still a slight negative pressure in the pleural space which sucks the water a little way up the glass tube in the drainage bottle. The fluid level should swing freely with the patient's breathing.

The drainage tubes from the patient to the bottles should be long enough to allow free movement both in bed and out of bed into a chair. The patient should be encouraged to move about as much as possible. The tubes should not be clamped during physiotherapy; care must be taken not to pull and disconnect them during movement nor to allow them to become kinked.

The tubes should be clamped during transit if for any reason one wishes to move the drainage bottles above the level of the patient to the opposite side of the bed. If a large air leak is present, the clamp should be released as quickly as possible.

If by accident a tube should become disconnected, the part connected to the patient should be clamped and reconnected to the drainage bottle immediately. The clamp should then be removed and the fluid level checked. If there is any cause for concern the medical staff should be informed.

If a patient has a persistent apical air pocket, and the drainage tube is still in place, it is sometimes helpful to give him breathing exercises (apical expansion) lying on his sound side with the bed elevated to about 18 in.

N.B. This system of drainage tubes does not apply to pneumonectomy cases (p. 51).

Intermittent Positive Pressure Breathing (IPPB)

If the patient retains secretions and is unable to breathe and cough effectively despite all methods described above, it might be necessary to combine treatment with IPPB to assist in better lung expansion and removal of secretions (p. 75). Pressure must be kept low (below 14 cm of water) to prevent any increase in air leak, and the treatment must only be given with the agreement of the surgeon concerned.

Naso-pharyngeal and naso-tracheal suction

If, after trying every other possible method, a patient is still unable to cough effectively

45

and has sputum retention, as a last resort it might be necessary to use naso-pharyngeal suction to stimulate coughing.

It must be emphasised that this is very rarely necessary and is unpleasant for the patient.

A catheter should be lubricated with a water-soluble jelly and gently passed through the nasal passage so that it curves down into the pharynx. If effective coughing is stimulated with the catheter in this position there is no need to proceed further. It is usually more effective to pass the catheter beyond the pharynx through the vocal cords and into the trachea. This is easiest to perform correctly if the head is in extension, and if the patient can co-operate, it is helpful if he puts out his tongue. The catheter should be slipped into the trachea during the phase of inspiration and efficient coughing is then stimulated. Further suction may be unnecessary once the patient has regained an effective cough.

During the first two post-operative days the patient should be encouraged to do his breathing exercises and coughing and leg movements for a few minutes at least every hour that he is awake. He should also practise his arm movements from time to time. It is valuable if the night nurse is able to remind the patient to take some deep breaths and to cough when she has to waken him for nursing purposes.

THIRD DAY AFTER OPERATION

The number of treatments are reduced according to the patient's condition; 3 or even 2 treatments will probably be sufficient but the patient must continue to practise his own exercises several times a day.

Treatment consists of:

1 Breathing exercises as above. These can be carried out sitting in a chair. As soon as unilateral expansion of the affected side is sufficiently good, bilateral basal expansion (p. 7) can be included (pneumonectomy excepted).

2 Effective coughing.

3 Postural drainage if necessary. Moderately vigorous activity, e.g. climbing stairs or walking immediately prior to postural drainage is helpful in loosening secretions by stimulating deeper breathing. Drainage is discontinued when the radiograph shows satisfactory re-expansion, and sputum has decreased.

4 Shoulder girdle and shoulder movements. Exercises should include active assisted movements through as full a range as possible. When the drainage tubes have been removed, full range of motion should be achieved.

5 Foot and leg exercises should be continued until the patient is walking around several times a day.

6 Posture should be corrected if necessary.

7 Simple trunk mobility exercises can be included if necessary.

8 Walking and increasing activity should be encouraged.

FOURTH DAY ONWARDS

Exercises as for the third day should be continued, but the number of sessions with the physiotherapist should be reduced as soon as possible. Walking upstairs should be introduced when the patient is fit enough. Controlled diaphragmatic breathing with walking should be taught when necessary.

BEFORE DISCHARGE

1 There should be good and equal movement on both sides of the chest (except following pneumonectomy).

2 Exercise tolerance should be restored to the extent that the patient can climb as many stairs as he has at home without becoming unduly breathless. After operations such as decortication of the lung and plication of bullae, exercise tolerance may be noticeably improved.

3 Full range movements should be restored to the shoulder joint and shoulder girdle.

4 Posture should be as good as preoperative posture.

The patient should continue breathing exercises for 3–4 weeks following the operation, although he will probably be discharged after 2–3 weeks. These should consist of localised expansion exercises to the appropriate areas to help in restoring maximum respiratory function and to prevent chest deformity.

PULMONARY SURGERY FOR INFANTS

Pulmonary surgery is rarely performed in infants, but when it is necessary the principles of physiotherapy are the same as for cardiac surgery (p. 64). Older children undergoing pulmonary surgery will be treated on the same lines as adults.

COMPLICATIONS OF PULMONARY SURGERY

1 Sputum retention

This is the most common complication of pulmonary surgery. If secretions are not removed, collapse of varying sized areas of lung tissue may follow. Physiotherapy is aimed at preventing this complication, but if it should occur intensive physiotherapy is essential (see previous section).

2 Persistent pneumothorax

If an air leak persists for more than forty-eight hours following surgery, an alveolar or bronchiolar leak should be suspected. The leak occurs from alveoli or bronchioli adjacent to the area of lung resected. A pneumothorax may be visible radiologically. Alveolar leaks heal quickly once the raw surface of lung comes against the chest wall, but bronchiolar leaks persist longer and may require resuturing.

It may be necessary to insert another tube if the drainage tube has already been removed and air is accumulating in the pleural cavity. If no drainage tube is in place, and the pneumothorax is increasing in size, a tension pneumothorax may develop, and physiotherapy should be discontinued until an intercostal tube has been reinserted.

If a pneumothorax is allowed to remain for a prolonged period, it is a potential source of infection and may result in an empyema. If a small pneumothorax is present (with or without a drainage tube in place), expansion exercises should be given, particularly over the apical area, and the patient should be instructed to hold full inspiration slightly longer than usual. In the case of a large apical pneumothorax (with a drainage tube in place) showing no signs of reduction in size, it is worth laying the patient on his unaffected side and raising the foot of the bed to a height of about 20 in (50 cm). In this position, expansion exercises for the apical area should be practised; this may assist in reduction of the air space.

3 Surgical emphysema

If air pressure builds up in the pleural space as a result of a communication between the lungs and pleura, air may track into the tissue layers producing what is known as surgical emphysema. A crackling sensation is apparent when the area is palpated. It usually starts around the site of a drainage tube or suture line and may spread into adjacent tissues causing swelling of the chest wall and neck, and extending in severe cases to the face and eyelids.

This condition usually subsides with correct tube management but the physiotherapist must take care not to aggravate the condition. During coughing the glottis is closed and the intrathoracic pressure raised; therefore more air is likely to escape into the tissues. Energetic coughing must be avoided if this is increasing the surgical emphysema. Loosening and removal of any bronchial secretions that are present must be assisted by deep breathing exercises and 'huffing', instead of coughing.

4 Bronchopleural fistula

A bronchopleural fistula is a communication between the bronchus and pleural cavity. This is a hazardous complication and usually occurs as a result of infection and disruption of the bronchial stump a week or ten days after pneumonectomy, or more rarely after lobectomy.

The signs of a fistula are: a sharp rise in pulse rate, swinging temperature, irritating cough and increase in sputum which may be blood-stained. This may be followed by the sudden expectoration of large amounts of fluid and eventually pus from the infected space.

Treatment consists of aspiration of infected fluid or the insertion of a drainage tube, instillation of antibiotics and postural drainage. Care must be taken to avoid infecting the remaining lung tissue. Resuturing of the bronchial stump may be necessary if healing does not occur. With bronchopleural fistula after pneumonectomy there is a serious risk of flooding the remaining lung with infected pleural fluid. It is essential that the physiotherapist keeps the remaining lung clear, and great care must be taken when positioning the patient to prevent any 'spill over' of fluid. The patient should always turn with the affected side at a lower level than the unaffected side.

Following lobectomy, both sides should be drained with the patient in the prone position in order to prevent any 'spill over'. Once the fluid has been drained by insertion of an intercostal tube, it may be safe to drain the remaining segments of the affected lung in the orthodox postural drainage positions. The affected side should be drained first, and the unaffected side drained afterwards in case there has been any 'spill over'.

5 Pleural effusion

A certain amount of blood-stained effusion always collects after resection, and the purpose of the basal tube is to drain this fluid. Aspiration may be necessary if fluid reaccumulates after removal of the drainage tube. If excessive fluid is allowed to remain, fibrin will be deposited on the visceral pleura causing thickening and restriction of movement. Expansion exercises should be given to the affected area.

6 Haemothorax

In rare cases, haemorrhage into the pleural cavity may occur. This is known as haemothorax. Re-operation may be necessary to seal off bleeding points and remove blood clot from the pleural cavity. Once bleeding has been controlled, breathing exercises should be given to avoid restriction of chest movement due to pleural thickening.

INDIVIDUAL SURGICAL CONDITIONS

Lobectomy

Resection of one or more lobes of a lung.

The pre- and post-operative treatment is as already described.

If the lobectomy is for bronchiectasis, postural drainage is an essential part of the treatment both before and after surgery.

After lobectomy there will be some displacement of the bronchi as the remaining lung expands to fill the space. One must therefore adjust postural drainage positions to find the optimal position for each individual patient.

A simple lobectomy may be performed for bronchial carcinoma, but if the neoplasm has spread into the main bronchus the surgeon may perform a *lobectomy by 'sleeve resection'*. This technique has been devised in order to clear as much tissue as possible into which the neoplasm may have spread, whilst preserving maximum lung function. An end-to-end anastomosis of the main bronchus with the lower lobe bronchus is performed after resecting the affected portion (fig. 44). The patient is more likely to have difficulty in clearing sputum after this type of operation as the anastomosis may be oedematous and partially occlude

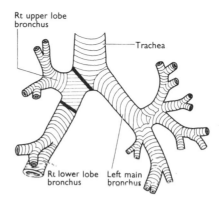

Fig. 44. *Lobectomy by sleeve resection.*

the airway. There may be some bleeding into the lower lobe causing thick blood-stained secretions. The principles and means of treatment are exactly the same as for a simple lobectomy.

If a bronchial neoplasm has invaded the chest wall, it may be necessary for the surgeon to perform a *lobectomy with partial resection of the chest wall*. In these cases paradoxical chest movement may occur. This is an indrawing of the resected area of chest wall during inspiration, and ballooning of the area on expiration. Breathing exercises become difficult and ineffective in these circumstances and a firm 'paradox pad' should be applied to the area to correct this movement. The pad should be made of cotton wool or similar material and be strapped firmly into position.

There is more pain than usual when a section of the chest wall is resected and therefore analgesia before physiotherapy is of particular importance.

Segmental resection

Removal of a segment of the lung.

A segmental resection may be performed to remove diseased areas of tuberculous lung tissue, non-malignant tumours or cysts.

The pre- and post-operative physiotherapy is the same as in the general description (p. 39). Although only a small area of lung tissue is removed, the adjoining lung may be affected by handling during the operation causing more secretions to form. There may be a larger air leak and more exudate draining from the pleural cavity after this operation than after a simple lobectomy. It is common to have persistent blood-stained sputum for at least a week after surgery.

Wedge resection

A very small area of lung is removed in order to resect small non-malignant tumours or cysts such as hamartoma, or small hydatid cysts. There is usually no problem with air leak or excessive exudate, but patients are likely to have a moderate amount of sputum.

Pneumonectomy

Total excision of one lung.

The extent of operation required for bronchial carcinoma is uncertain until the thorax has been opened and this has already been discussed (p. 40). There are other conditions such as tuberculosis or bronchiectasis for which a pneumonectomy may be necessary. If a patient is definitely scheduled for a pneumonectomy, the physiotherapist can be more precise in pre-operative instructions.

PRE-OPERATIVE TRAINING

This should include:

1 Explanation.
2 Removal of secretions if present.

3 Breathing exercises.
(a) Diaphragmatic breathing.
(b) Lateral basal expansion for the unaffected side.
4 'Huffing' to loosen secretions.
5 Effective coughing.
6 Foot and leg exercises.
7 Posture.
8 Arm and shoulder girdle movements.

POST-OPERATIVE TREATMENT

The treatment is essentially the same as that described previously (p. 43). The following points should be noted:
1 Some patients find difficulty in coughing and tend to strain. It is important to avoid straining during coughing owing to the risk of breakdown of the bronchial suture line and resultant bronchopleural fistula. Patients should therefore loosen the secretions by correct breathing exercises and 'huffing'.
2 If postural drainage is necessary, the patient should lie as far over on to the operated side as possible, supported by pillows and with the foot of the bed raised.

A large defect in the pericardial wall may have been left, and under some circumstances the heart can herniate through this defect into the pleural cavity, and this distortion of the heart and great vessels can cause shock. The institution of postural drainage following a radical pneumonectomy should therefore be discussed with the surgeon concerned.
3 The patient should not lie on the unaffected side for at least two weeks after the operation, i.e. until fibrin has formed in the pneumonectomy space, and the danger of bronchopleural fistula has passed.
4 Bilateral basal expansion exercises may be started at the end of the first week to prevent future flattening and rigidity of the

chest wall. Equal movement should obviously not be expected.

5 The patient normally sits in a chair for varying periods within twenty-four hours of the operation, and walks within two or three days. If the post-operative progress is satisfactory, walking on the stairs can be started within one week, but this depends on the condition of each individual patient. Controlled breathing with walking, on the level and up stairs, should be taught if the patient is dyspnoeic on exertion.

DRAINAGE TUBE

Some surgeons leave a drainage tube in the pleural cavity connected to an underwater seal, for approximately twenty-four hours. This tube remains clamped, and is only released for approximately one minute every hour according to instructions. Suction is never applied.

The function of this tube is to control the amount of fluid remaining in the pneumonectomy space, and thereby prevent mediastinal shift. If there is too much fluid in the space, there is a shift of the mediastinum towards the remaining lung causing pressure on, and partial collapse of the lung. The patient becomes breathless, and may develop cardiac arrhythmias due to disturbance of the heart and great vessels in the mediastinum.

If there is too little fluid in the space, the mediastinum shifts away from the remaining lung and again arrhythmias may occur. There will also be over-inflation of the remaining lung.

Deviation of the trachea indicates mediastinal shift; this will be confirmed radiologically. In order to correct this, it may be necessary for the surgeon to aspirate the hemithorax and adjust the pressures with a Maxwell Box. By this means air can either be withdrawn or instilled.

Some surgeons like to adjust the fluid level in the hemithorax by routine aspiration so that it is below the level of the bronchial stump, until the danger of bronchopleural fistula has passed.

COMPLICATIONS FOLLOWING PNEUMONECTOMY

1 *Injury to recurrent laryngeal nerve*

During radical pneumonectomy, the left recurrent laryngeal nerve is sometimes damaged, or may even have to be resected. This results in inability to close the vocal cords and therefore partial loss of effective coughing power. The patient may be able to clear his secretions adequately by breathing exercises and 'huffing', but the addition of IPPB (intermittent positive pressure breathing) is often helpful, if the surgeon gives permission. Pressure must be kept low, i.e. no higher than 10 cm H_2O.

2 *Phrenic nerve paralysis*

If a tumour involves the phrenic nerve, it may be necessary to resect it causing paralysis of the diaphragm on the affected side. The patient will have an ineffective cough due to the paradoxical movement of the diaphragm. IPPB is helpful in these cases to aerate the lung more efficiently if the surgeon gives permission.

3 *Bronchopleural fistula* (p. 48)

Thoracotomy for inoperable bronchial carcinoma

The surgeon may find on opening the thorax that the neoplasm has invaded vital organs, or is so extensive as to make lobectomy or pneumonectomy impossible. In this case the thorax is closed leaving one tube in the pleural space to drain the post-operative exudate.

Post-operative physiotherapy is the same as for lobectomy. The clearance of secretions may be made difficult if the tumour causes distortion and obstruction of the airways. The physiotherapist should bear in mind the general condition of the patient and should make every effort to clear the bronchial secretions without causing the patient undue distress. A few patients with inoperable carcinoma deteriorate rapidly, and undue pressure should not be brought to bear on the patient if physiotherapy does not relieve his symptoms.

Insertion of radioactive gold grains

When a tumour has been found to be inoperable by resection, the surgeon may implant radioactive gold grains to assist destruction of the growth. This treatment is used in certain cases as an alternative to radiotherapy.

The pre- and post-operative physiotherapy is the same as that for lobectomy.

Post-operatively there is a limit to the time the physiotherapist may stay in the patient's room due to the radio-activity. She must carefully divide her time to allow a few short treatments in the day, or ideally share the treatments with another physiotherapist. The maximum time allowed will increase each day. A monitoring badge should be worn.

The chest radiographs may show gross shadowing due to the radio-activity. Two or three days after surgery, sputum may increase and contain necrotic material.

Plication of emphysematous bullae

If large emphysematous bullae are occupying much space in the thoracic cavity, the surgeon may perform a thoracotomy to tie off these bullae so that the normal lung tissue can expand into the area previously occupied by the cysts. Lung function will be improved as a result.

Instruction in diaphragmatic breathing with relaxation and control of the upper chest is very important. The patients undergoing this operation usually have severe respiratory disability and therefore may experience distress and difficulty in expectoration during the first few post-operative days, and probably require intensive physiotherapy with the use of intermittent positive pressure breathing. Apical breathing is unnecessary as the emphysematous patient will already be over-inflating the upper chest. Walking with controlled breathing on the level and going upstairs should be taught.

Pleurectomy

A pleurectomy may be performed if a patient suffers from recurrent pneumothoraces. A small thoracotomy incision is made and the parietal pleura is stripped off the lateral chest wall. As the lung re-expands, adhesions form between the chest wall and visceral pleura, preventing recurrence of pneumothorax. Blebs or bullae may be oversewn at the same time.

The basic treatment previously described is suitable, emphasising basal and apical expansion exercises for the affected side. If a drainage tube is in place pre-operatively to deal with the spontaneous pneumothorax, 'huffing' and coughing can be taught in the usual way. If, however, there is a partial pneumothorax and no tube is in place, 'huffing' and coughing should be demonstrated only. Vigorous coughing might cause an increase in the size of the pneumothorax.

There are unlikely to be excessive secretions post-operatively when the operation has been performed for idiopathic spontaneous pneumothorax, as there is usually no underlying lung disease. Emphasis must be on expansion exercises.

If, however, the operation has been performed on a patient suffering from cystic fibrosis where spontaneous pneumothorax occurs due to cyst formation, there will be a definite problem with sticky secretions. Postural drainage must be started on the first day post-operatively and performed at least four times a day.

Decortication of the lung

If the pleura has become thickened and fibrosed following empyema (tuberculous or non-tuberculous), or haemothorax, the surgeon may perform a thoracotomy and strip off the thickened layers of pleura. If simpler measures have failed to eliminate an empyema cavity, this operation may consist of complete pleurectomy with excision of the empyema cavity. The lung is then free to fill the space formerly occupied by the empyema.

The basic physiotherapy for any thoracotomy applies. Pre-operatively, movement of the chest over the affected area may be very limited, and there may be dramatic improvement after decortication. Rapid expansion of the lung is essential; this is achieved by applying strong suction to the drainage tubes, and vigorous breathing exercises. Basal and apical expansion exercises must be emphasised, and belt exercises may be necessary to encourage expansion in the later stages of treatment (see p. 8).

In patients with extensive tuberculous scarring, the lung may fail to fill the hemithorax completely at the end of the operation. The surgeon may then have to consider thoracoplasty at a later date to obliterate the air space.

Thoracoplasty

This operation is now rarely required because of advances in the treatment of tuberculosis. It was used formerly as a means of producing permanent collapse of diseased lung tissue so that healing could take place. Nowadays it may be used occasionally to obliterate a space in the thoracic cavity; for example in chronic empyema or following resection of lung tissue.

During surgery several ribs are resected subperiosteally. For extensive thoracoplasty, up to 8 ribs, including the first, may be resected; this is often carried out in two stages. When the operation is performed to obliterate a space, the first rib is not usually removed and the neck remains more stable because the scalene muscles retain their insertion.

An unsightly scoliosis will occur if correct physiotherapy is not carried out. It is vital that the patient is aware of the deformity likely to occur, and be able to correct it.

PRE-OPERATIVE TRAINING

1. *Breathing exercises*

Diaphragmatic breathing, unilateral basal expansion for the affected side, and effective coughing should be taught. The patient should be shown how to support the apical area of his chest when he coughs.

2. *Postural correction in front of a mirror*

The patient will tend to develop a scoliosis with the concavity in the cervical spine and the convexity in the thoracic spine on the side of the operation (fig. 45). He must be taught how to correct these tendencies by means of lateral movement of the neck towards the side of the thoracoplasty, depression of the shoulder girdle on the operation side and correct alignment of the shoulders and pelvis.

3. Retraction of the scapulae should be taught, also full-range arm movements on the side of the thoracoplasty.

POST-OPERATIVE TREATMENT

Day of operation

Treatment is started as soon as the patient has recovered consciousness and consists of assisted coughing with firm support over

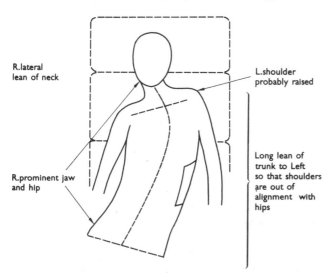

R.lateral lean of neck

L.shoulder probably raised

R.prominent jaw and hip

Long lean of trunk to Left so that shoulders are out of alignment with hips

Fig. 45. *Postural defects likely after a left thoracoplasty (front view).*

54

the apical region of the chest wall, diaphragmatic breathing and localised basal expansion on the operation side. If there is paradoxical movement of the chest wall, a firm pad should be applied below the clavicle extending down into the axilla; it should be rebandaged regularly until the paradox has disappeared.

This is very painful operation and adequate analgesia must be given before physiotherapy.

1st Day

1 Arrange the pillows comfortably.
2 Correct posture, without a mirror at this stage as it may be demoralising for the patient.
3 Diaphragmatic breathing.
4 Localised basal expansion on the affected side.
5 Assisted coughing with firm support.
6 Active assisted arm movements; these are often more easily performed with a flexed elbow against resistance.
7 Depression of the shoulder girdle on the thoracoplasty side.
8 Neck lateral lean towards the thoracoplasty side; it may be helpful to give resistance below the mastoid process.

2nd Day

1 As above, but if the patient is looking better a mirror may be used.
2 Increased resistance can be used for arm movements.
3 Retraction of the scapulae.
4 Extra neck movements are included: side-flexion towards the operation side only, forward flexion and rotation.

The exercises are gradually progressed with the patient performing them sitting upright, then standing. Trunk forward flexion and side-flexion may be started after about 1 week. Trunk rotation is delayed until about 3 weeks after the operation.

Breathing exercises may be discontinued after about 10 days if there are no pulmonary complications, but postural exercises are progressed and continued until the patient is discharged from hospital. Many patients are able to maintain a good posture when standing still but not when walking, and their attention must be drawn to this. When discharged from hospital, the patient is advised to continue his exercises and posture correction, until 3 months after the date of his operation.

TWO STAGE THORACOPLASTY

If the operation is performed in two stages, treatment is progressed as for the first stage, but the patients often have more difficulty in moving the arm. On very rare occasions the scapula is tucked in behind the 8th rib and it is wiser to delay arm elevation until after the third day.

Surgery for diaphragmatic hernia, achalasia of the cardia (Heller's operation), oesophagectomy, ruptured oesophagus

The same principles of physiotherapy before and after surgery apply for these conditions. A lateral thoracotomy through the sixth or seventh intercostal space is used and these lower incisions are usually more painful than the higher ones. Diaphragmatic breathing and unilateral basal expansion must be emphasised.

After surgery for diaphragmatic hernia, coughing should not be forced during the first few days.

Patients undergoing surgery of the oesophagus should not be given postural drainage unless absolutely essential, as this may cause regurgitation of the gastric juices.

Correction of pectus excavatum

Pectus excavatum, or funnel chest, is a deformity where there is undue depression of the sternum. It may be corrected surgically if it is causing either diminished lung function or cosmetic problems. The aim of the operation is to hold the sternum forward. Various techniques are used and the majority of patients have a median sternotomy.

Pre-operatively unilateral basal expansion exercises for both sides of the chest are practised. Post-operatively the surgeon probably requires the patient to lie flat for at least twenty-four hours. He should not be nursed in a semi-recumbent position. He should either lie flat or sit in an upright chair out of bed. Breathing exercises must be practised immediately post-operatively. The commencement of arm and trunk movements and ambulation must be discussed with the surgeon. Shoulder girdle exercises and posture correction will be necessary as soon as permission is given.

Thymectomy

Thymectomy is performed for removal of thymoma often associated with myasthenia gravis. The incision is usually a high median sternotomy.

The basic principles of pre- and post-operative physiotherapy apply, but patients with myasthenia gravis become easily fatigued, and the physiotherapist should take care not to tire them. If possible, treatment should be given soon after the administration of prostigmin.

Some myasthenic patients require ventilation post-operatively and often suffer from excessive secretions which occur as a side-effect of prostigmin. Prolonged treatment cannot be tolerated and occasionally it may be necessary to cease treatment before the chest has been completely cleared in order to prevent fatigue (p. 66 for ventilator treatment).

CARDIAC SURGERY

Most open heart operations are performed through an incision known as a median sternotomy. These include: valve replacements, valve annuloplasty, open mitral or pulmonary valvotomy, closure of atrial or ventricular septal defect, Mustard's procedure for transposition of the great vessels, total correction of Fallot's tetralogy, correction of anomalous pulmonary venous drainage, excision of ventricular or aortic aneurysm, saphenous-coronary graft, removal of cardiac myxoma. Pulmonary embolectomy can be included as cardio-pulmonary bypass is also necessary for this operation.

Some surgeons prefer to perform mitral valve replacement, mitral valve annuloplasty, and closure of atrial septal defect through a right postero-lateral incision.

For most closed heart operations a lateral thoracotomy is used. These include: mitral valvotomy, ligation of patent ductus arteriosus, atrial septectomy, banding of the pulmonary artery, shunt-anastomoses for Fallot's tetralogy and excision of coarctation of the aorta.

A median sternotomy, or possibly bilateral anterior thoracotomy, will be used for pericardiectomy.

The physiotherapist should know which incision the surgeon will use for each patient in order that emphasis can be laid on the exercises that will be most important during the post-operative period.

With cardiac patients, it is essential to adapt treatment to each individual's condition. A strict routine cannot be followed and it is vital never to exhaust a patient. Pre-operative training is just as important as it is for those patients undergoing pulmonary surgery. It should be started as early as possible, preferably at least five days before surgery.

Aims of physiotherapy following cardiac surgery

1 To preserve adequate ventilation.
2 To assist with removal of excessive secretions in the airways.
3 To assist the circulation in the legs and thereby help to prevent post-operative venous thrombosis.
4 To maintain mobility of the shoulders, shoulder girdle and spine.
5 To prevent postural defects.
6 To restore exercise tolerance.

PRE-OPERATIVE TRAINING

1 Explanation to the patient

Explanation by the physiotherapist, in order to gain the patient's confidence and co-operation, should be similar to that described for pulmonary surgery (p. 39).

The importance of maintaining adequate

ventilation of the lungs by deep breathing and the clearance of excessive secretions from the airways must be explained. Reassurance should be given that deep breathing, coughing and moving around in bed will do no harm to the stitches, drainage tubes or operation site.

A doctor should tell the patient about the operation, including the position of drainage tubes, intravenous drip, nasogastric tube, urine catheter, electrocardiograph leads and the probability that he will need an endotracheal tube and the use of a ventilator for a few hours post-operatively. The patient should be warned that if he wakes up with an endotracheal tube in place, speaking will be temporarily impossible, but the staff will be able to understand his requirements.

The physiotherapist can describe the treatment to be performed if artificial ventilation is likely, or alternatively she can explain that breathing exercises will not be started until the endotracheal tube has been removed.

2 Removal of secretions

The majority of patients about to undergo cardiac surgery will have clear lungs and will not need assistance to clear the airways. There are, however, some patients with severe mitral valve disease or long-standing pulmonary hypertension who may have developed associated chronic obstructive lung disease, and in such cases assistance with removal of secretions is required. In the earlier stage of cardiac disease the patient may have a persistent dry cough or expectorate frothy white sputum. This is not a problem that can be dealt with by physiotherapy.

If a patient has a cold or other respiratory tract infection, surgery will almost certainly be postponed until the chest is clear.

If a chronic bronchitic is to undergo cardiac surgery he may need assistance to clear excessive secretions from his airways. A modified form of postural drainage (p. 11), combined with breathing exercises, should be used. Care should be taken not to cause undue fatigue or dyspnoea.

The head-down postural drainage position should never be used for cardiac patients before or after surgery unless specifically requested by the surgeon concerned, because of the risk of precipitating pulmonary oedema.

3 Breathing exercises

(a) DIAPHRAGMATIC BREATHING (p. 5)

This exercise assists the loosening of secretions by aerating the lower areas of the lungs. In order to perform this exercise correctly, encouragement must be given to relax the upper chest and shoulder girdle. If a patient suffers from severe dyspnoea, relaxation and breathing control may be found easier in the high side-lying position.

(b) UNILATERAL BASAL EXPANSION (p. 6)

For patients having a median sternotomy, expansion of both bases will be inhibited after surgery, and therefore unilateral expansion of both lung bases should be practised in the half-lying position. Expansion for the side of the incision must be emphasised when a lateral thoracotomy is to be used.

Holding full inspiration for one or two

seconds during each breath taken is useful in assisting aeration of the alveoli.

Pre-operatively, the patient should be encouraged to practise these exercises three or four times during the day. He should understand that for the first two or three days after the operation he should practise deep breathing for at least a few minutes every hour that he is awake, and not only when visited by the physiotherapist.

4 Effective coughing

Effective 'huffing' and coughing is taught as for pulmonary surgery (p. 41). The physiotherapist should show the patient how she will support the chest over the incision, and how he can support it himself. For a median sternotomy the patient can hold his hands directly over the front of the sternum (fig. 46) or fold his arms across the chest giving lateral support as well as pressure of the forearms anteriorly; alternatively he can hold a pillow against the

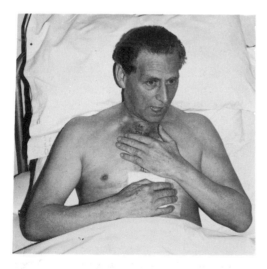

Fig. 46. *Median sternotomy supported by patient.*

anterior part of his chest. For a lateral incision the arm of the unaffected side is placed across the front of the chest, the hand giving pressure just below the incision, the other elbow giving pressure inwards to the chest wall (fig. 41).

5 Foot and leg exercises

All patients are taught simple foot exercises and knee flexion and extension in order to assist the circulation, and help prevent post-operative venous thrombosis. The importance of practising these movements several times during every waking hour after surgery should be stressed.

6 Posture, shoulder girdle and arm movements

The habitual posture of the patient is noted pre-operatively, also his range of arm movements. Those patients having a median sternotomy are unlikely to have difficulty with shoulder movements after surgery, but the shoulder girdle may become stiff and many patients tend to adopt a slightly kyphotic posture. Shoulder shrugging and 'shrug-circling' are useful exercises and can be practised briefly pre-operatively.

Patients having a lateral thoracotomy need arm and shoulder girdle exercises, and postural correction similarly to those undergoing pulmonary surgery (p. 42).

7 Pre-operative observations

During pre-operative instruction the physiotherapist should note the patient's normal chest movement, his exercise tolerance, and his habitual sleeping position, for example using several pillows. The latter is important not only because of the patient's possible orthopnoea but also because these patients will need reassurance should it be necessary to lay them flat in the post-operative phase.

POST-OPERATIVE TREATMENT

Before treatment the physiotherapist must read the operation notes, and the report of the patient's progress since the operation. Several quick observations must be made:

1 Respiration: is the patient being artificially ventilated? If not, what is the respiratory rate?
2 Level of consciousness: is the patient alert and fully responsive? Has he moved all his limbs to command since the operation?
3 Colour: is the patient cyanosed?
4 Blood pressure: has it been stable since the operation?
5 Pulse and temperature.
6 ECG: has the cardiac rhythm been stable, or have there been arrhythmias?
7 Pacemaker: is the heart being artificially paced?
8 Drugs: are drugs required to maintain a reasonable blood pressure? What time was the last dose of analgesic given?
9 Drains: where were the drainage tubes inserted at operation? Was the pleural cavity on either side of the chest opened?
10 Drainage: has there been excessive bleeding from any drain site?
11 Blood gas results: is the arterial oxygen tension unduly low or the carbon dioxide level unduly high?
12 Chest radiograph.
13 Sputum: what colour sputum and what quantity has (a) been sucked from the endotracheal tube if ventilated, or (b) been expectorated by the patient?

14 Urine output: has the patient been passing urine since the operation?

Observations of this nature should be made by the physiotherapist before every treatment, and any change in the general condition should be taken into account.

DAY OF OPERATION

If the patient is not on a ventilator, breathing exercises can be started on the day of the operation (provided the cardiovascular system is stable) as soon as he is conscious enough to co-operate. After some deep breathing exercises, attempts at 'huffing' and coughing should be made.

FIRST AND SECOND DAYS AFTER OPERATION

Physiotherapy will probably be necessary four times during the day. The length of treatment should be modified according to the patient's condition and should not cause undue fatigue.

1 Ventilator treatment

The majority of patients undergoing open heart surgery receive intermittent positive pressure ventilation via an endotracheal tube during the first post-operative night. If there are excessive secretions in the lungs it may be wise to give physiotherapy before the anaesthetist removes the endotracheal tube. The doctor in charge must advise on this matter.

The indications for physiotherapy depend not only on the secretions in the lungs: at this stage the state of the circulation and the arterial oxygen tension (P_aO_2) are much more important. Treatment with manual hyperinflation of the lungs and gentle chest vibrations (p. 66) may be indicated, but it is probably better not employed as a routine in cardiac surgical patients. Indications for its use are the presence of well-defined areas of localised pulmonary collapse, or evidence of secretions which cannot be readily mobilised with routine suction.

Manual hyperinflation and chest vibrations can be very effective in aiding removal of secretions but it may be contra-indicated since it can cause a drop in cardiac output, fall in blood pressure and sometimes a drop in P_aO_2. It should therefore be prescribed on an individual basis, the decision largely depending on the relative requirements of the circulatory and respiratory symptoms.

If the cardiovascular state is unstable, efficient endotracheal suction would probably be adequate to maintain reasonably clear lungs until the general condition warrants more energetic treatment.

If, however, excessive secretions are present, the physiotherapist can perform gentle vibrations in time with the normal expiratory phase of the ventilator. This is often a less efficient method of treatment, but a suitable compromise if the cardiovascular system is not yet stable enough to justify hyperinflation.

Many patients who have undergone cardiac surgery have very few secretions in their chest and need no physiotherapy at this stage.

2 Breathing exercises

If the patient is not being artificially ventilated, and his cardiovascular state is sufficiently stable, breathing exercises should be carried out. Those who have been ventilated should also start breathing exercises once the endotracheal tube has been removed. The patient should be sitting up in bed with the whole spine supported by pillows, so that diaphragmatic and chest movements are not inhibited.

Exercises should consist of:
(a) Diaphragmatic breathing.
(b) Unilateral basal expansion for both sides of the chest.

If there is a median sternotomy, expansion of both bases (unilaterally) must be encouraged. If a pleural drain is *in situ*, pain may limit movement and emphasis should be given to expand that side of the chest. With a lateral thoracotomy, emphasis must be given to expansion of the incision side.

If pain is severely limiting the respiratory excursion, the physiotherapist should arrange to treat the patient after an analgesic has been administered.

The patient should be reminded to take some deep breaths at least every hour whilst awake.

3 Coughing

Effective 'huffing' and coughing, as taught pre-operatively, must be encouraged with the chest firmly supported. The patient often finds it easier to cough when sitting forward in bed away from the pillows. Great care must be taken to avoid displacing any drips or wires attached to the patient.

In the absence of heart failure or co-existent lung disease, there are likely to be fewer secretions in the airways than after lung surgery, because the pleurae have often not been opened, and the lungs have not been handled.

If the air entry to the lungs is satisfactory, the chest radiograph reasonably clear and the patient is breathing efficiently, it will be unnecessary to turn him into the side-lying position. If there are secretions in the lungs that he is unable to clear, he should, with the doctor's permission, be positioned on his side, and breathing exercises should be carried out, followed by coughing.

The foot of the bed should never be raised for postural drainage of a cardiac patient unless it is specifically ordered by the surgeon.

If the patient is exhausted, and unable to breathe effectively, the gas exchange in the alveoli will be inefficient, and there may be retention of secretions. Physiotherapy in conjunction with an intermittent positive pressure breathing machine can help to improve the gas exchange and loosen secretions (p. 71). This is often effective in the sitting position, but may be used in side-lying if necessary.

4   Foot and leg exercises

The exercises taught pre-operatively should be practised, and the patient should be reminded to do these movements 5–10 times every hour that he is awake.

5   Shoulder movements

With a lateral thoracotomy it is important to start arm movements on the first post-operative day. With a median sternotomy these need not be started until the second day.

THIRD DAY ONWARDS

Treatment following cardiac surgery must be adapted to each individual patient's condition. The patient will start sitting out of bed any time after the first twenty-four hours according to his progress and the surgeon's wishes; and similarly, walking around the ward may be started as soon as the second or third post-operative day.

The number of times a day that physiotherapy is required depends on the patient's condition, and it can probably be reduced gradually to one or two treatments per day by the end of the first week.

Treatment should consist of:

1   Breathing exercises (as above). The patient can be positioned in side-lying if expansion is limited or air entry reduced. Bilateral basal expansion can be included.

2   Coughing, if secretions are present in the lungs.

3   Foot and leg exercises until the patient is walking in the ward several times a day.

4   Arm and shoulder girdle exercises.

5   Postural correction and gentle trunk exercises if necessary.

6   With the surgeon's permission, walking up the stairs can usually be started about 10 days from the time of operation. After cardiac surgery most patients find climbing stairs much less exhausting than pre-operatively, but on occasions it is helpful to teach controlled breathing with walking on the stairs.

Treatment must be modified if any complications occur.

BEFORE DISCHARGE

1   There should be good and equal movement on both sides of the chest.

2   There should be full range movements of the shoulder joints and shoulder girdle.

3   Posture should be as good as the pre-operative posture.

4   The patient should be able to climb as many stairs as he has at home without becoming breathless.

The patient should continue breathing exercises for 3–4 weeks following the operation, although he will probably be discharged after 2–3 weeks.

COMPLICATIONS OF CARDIAC SURGERY

Following cardiac surgery, the patient will be continuously assessed by the medical staff so that any complications may be detected and appropriate treatment prescribed. Such complications include: cardiac failure, tamponade, haemorrhage, arrhythmias, and fluid and electrolyte imbalance. Other complications that particularly influence the treatment given by the physiotherapist are as follows:

1 Pulmonary oedema

If a patient develops acute pulmonary oedema and is being artificially ventilated, physiotherapy should be temporarily discontinued until the condition has been treated. If the patient is breathing independently, he may require assistance to expectorate the excessive secretions, but medical treatment (diuretics, etc.) will be required to relieve the condition. Copious frothy sputum may be an indication of pulmonary oedema. This may be white at first, becoming pink if the condition is allowed to progress.

2 Pulmonary dysfunction after bypass surgery

After open heart surgery, areas of 'bronchial breathing' are often detected on auscultation. These are areas of collapse which may not be visible radiologically, and not necessarily due to retained secretions. This results in a lowering of the P_aO_2, unless the patient is breathing oxygen.

The aetiology of this abnormality is not completely understood, but it is probably due to several factors connected with the use of cardio-pulmonary bypass.

The physiotherapist should encourage deep breathing exercises and, if necessary, use IPPB to assist in opening up these areas of collapsed alveoli.

3 Compression of the left main bronchus

A grossly enlarged heart may compress the left main bronchus causing collapse of the left lower lobe. If this situation occurs, the patient should not be turned on to his left side as this can increase the compression.

4 Pleural effusion

Expansion exercises must be practised in order to prevent restriction of lung movement due to thickening of the pleura. Aspiration may be needed for large effusions.

5 Breakdown of the sternal sutures

If the sternal suture line is breaking down due to infection, the patient's temperature may be raised; there may be oozing from the wound, and possibly a noticeable 'click' when the patient coughs or breathes deeply. Firm support must be given to the chest during 'huffing' and coughing, both by the staff, and also by the patient when he is coughing independently. Care must be taken to prevent straining the suture line when the patient turns in bed.

6 Neurological damage

Occasionally, during cardiac surgery, the brain may be damaged by embolism or anoxia. The physiotherapist must treat any form of paralysis that occurs, and rehabilitate the patient as soon as possible. Obviously the patient's cardiac state may limit the form of rehabilitation to some extent.

7 Renal failure

Another rare complication of cardiac surgery is renal failure. Occasionally peritoneal dialysis will have to be instituted. Breathing exercises are particularly important to maintain function of the lung bases. Physiotherapy should be carried out during the period when the peritoneum is almost empty, in order to allow maximum basal expansion. The diaphragmatic action will be limited when the abdomen is filled with fluid, and the patient will find it uncomfortable if physiotherapy is given at this time.

PROBLEMS WITH INDIVIDUAL CARDIAC OPERATIONS

Resection of coarctation of the aorta

During the first ten days after resection of coarctation of the aorta, there are likely to be episodes of hypertension. The reason for this phenomenon is unknown, but if it occurs it could put a strain on the aortic suture line. The physiotherapist should be aware of the possibility and modify the treatment to avoid increasing the hypertension. It may be contra-indicated to lay the patient flat, even if bronchial secretions are present.

Pulmonary embolectomy

Pulmonary embolectomy may be performed

for massive pulmonary embolism. Post-operative physiotherapy should be along the same lines as for any open heart operation, but pulmonary dysfunction is especially common owing to the presence of small infarcts. The patient is likely to be cyanosed, and will expectorate old blood-stained sputum.

Manual hyperinflation with chest vibration may be indicated while the patient is artificially ventilated.

Pericardiectomy

Following this operation the patients are often troubled with excessive amounts of frothy sputum and need particular encouragement with coughing. Otherwise, the treatment is the same as for any closed heart operation.

Insertion of pacemaker

Pacemakers are inserted for the treatment of heart block. The incision used varies with the type of pacemaker, and the preference of the surgeon concerned; it may be an abdominal incision, lateral thoracotomy, or an axillary incision. Many elderly people undergo this operation, and although it is a relatively minor procedure, and the pleura is not opened, the physiotherapist must give pre- and post-operative treatment to prevent any chest complications.

CARDIAC SURGERY FOR CHILDREN

PRE-OPERATIVE TRAINING

The amount of pre-operative training possible in children naturally depends on their age. As well as teaching the child, it is important to explain the necessity of the exercises to the parents who are often with the children for long periods of the day and can encourage practice.

18 months–3 years

It is usually possible to teach deep breathing by means of blowing bubbles or paper tissues. If bronchial secretions are present pre-operatively, postural drainage can probably be performed (with the doctor's permission) and percussion over the chest usually induces coughing.

3 years upwards

Diaphragmatic breathing, localised basal expansion exercises and coughing can be taught. Possibly up to the age of 5, the incentive of blowing bubbles or paper tissues may be necessary. Postural drainage can be performed if required.

Arm movements can be encouraged by clapping the hands over the head, and for children of over 5 years old, more shoulder girdle and arm exercises can be included.

POST-OPERATIVE TREATMENT

The child may be in the side-lying position, and if a lateral incision has been used, gentle pressure can be given over the affected side to encourage expansion of the chest.

Spontaneous coughing is often induced with crying, but if the breath sounds are diminished, if secretions are present, and the child will not cough spontaneously, some other means of stimulating a cough must be used. The child can be 'tipped' if the doctor gives permission. Intermittent tracheal pressure is a means of stimulating the cough reflex by pressing laterally on the trachea with the finger tips. In children, the trachea is soft and mobile, pressure can produce apposition of the tracheal walls and instant stimulation of the cough reflex results. Naso-phrayngeal suction may be necessary if all else fails.

If one side of the chest is expanding poorly, the child should be encouraged to lie in bed on the opposite side.

Small children are often allowed up to run around the ward a day or two after surgery; this is the best way to stimulate deep breathing.

Many children have no problems with chest secretions after cardiac surgery, but some may develop very poor posture and are reluctant to move the affected shoulder, in which case suitable exercises must be given.

CARDIAC SURGERY FOR INFANTS

PRE-OPERATIVE TREATMENT

Infants with cardiac defects often suffer from pulmonary hypertension, and frequently have excessive secretions and are prone to repeated chest infections. It may be necessary to give physiotherapy pre-operatively to clear the chest. This consists of modified postural drainage, gentle vibrations and naso-pharyngeal suction to stimulate coughing.

POST-OPERATIVE TREATMENT

If the infant is artificially ventilated, physiotherapy may be requested by the doctor. Gentle chest vibrations and suction are given in a side-lying position, if possible. Manual hyperinflation with chest vibration may possibly be indicated (p. 68).

If the infant is not on a ventilator and excessive secretions are present in the chest, physiotherapy consists of gentle vibrations and naso-pharyngeal suction in the side-lying position. It is important that secretions do not become thick and occlude the small airways, therefore many infants are nursed in high humidity for the immediate post-operative period.

6 Physiotherapy for patients receiving mechanical assistance

INTERMITTENT POSITIVE PRESSURE VENTILATION (IPPV)

When a patient is being artificially ventilated via a tracheostomy or endotracheal tube, there are several factors, apart from the underlying disease, that predispose to excessive bronchial secretions and chest infection. These include:

1 The inability to cough effectively.

2 The absence of the normal deep sigh mechanism.

3 The presence of a tube which irritates the mucous membrane.

4 The tendency for drying and crusting of secretions, and infection, due to bypass of the upper respiratory tract.

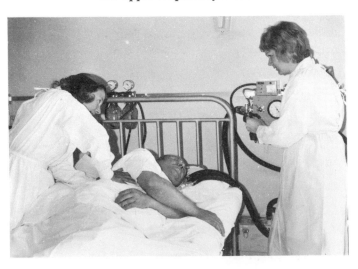

Fig. 47. *Manual hyperinflation with vibrations.*

By adequate humidification and tracheal suction, and care in maintaining sterile precautions, problems of excessive secretions can be kept to a minimum. However, assistance with removal of secretions is often required and the most effective method is known as manual hyperinflation with chest vibration. It is often termed 'bag squeezing', but this name does not infer the all important type of inflation that is given.

Technique

The patient is positioned on his side if possible, and the tracheostomy tube, or endotracheal tube, is disconnected from the ventilator and connected to a manual inflation bag. One person, usually an anaesthetist, squeezes the bag, inflating the chest with a slow deep inspiration which promotes complete aeration of the alveoli. After holding the full inspiration momentarily, the bag is released quickly, to allow a high expiratory flow rate. The physiotherapist has her hands on the side of the lower rib cage, and starts to compress the chest just at the end of the inspiratory period, fractionally before the bag is released. This accurate synchronisation between the two operators is essential to produce the best effect. The chest compression reinforcing the high expiratory flow rate from the bag, assists movement of the secretions in the periphery of the lung towards the main airways (fig. 47).

Approximately six deep breaths with chest vibrations are given, starting at the lung base; this is followed by suction performed by the nurse. If the patient is

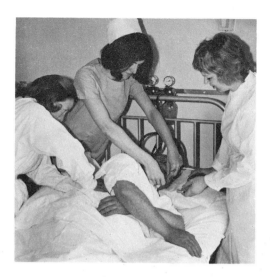

Fig. 48. *Tracheal suction with vibrations.*

conscious and able to co-operate he is encouraged to attempt to cough actively when the suction catheter has been inserted, and at the same time the physiotherapist vibrates the chest to assist removal of secretions (fig. 48).

The whole procedure is probably repeated two or three times with the physiotherapist vibrating over the basal area. When that area is clear, the middle and upper areas of the chest are treated if secretions are present.

Frequency

The number of times per day that treatment is performed depends both on the condition of the patient's chest and on his general condition. It may be necessary to carry it out every two hours, or even hourly, or it may only be required once or twice a day. Where possible, treatment should be timed to coincide with the nurses turning regime to avoid unnecessary discomfort to the patient.

Thick secretions

If the secretions are thick, it is often helpful to insert 2 or 3 ml of normal saline (0·9%) into the trachea before hyperinflating the chest. The saline will go into the most dependent bronchi, and should therefore be inserted before turning the patient or laying him down to drain the affected area.

Equipment for inflation

There are many types of bag available for lung inflation; either the rebreathing bag attached to a ventilator may be used, or a separate hand ventilation system. It is important that the system provides a good elastic recoil when the bag is released. A 2-litre bag is normally used.

Most commonly a mixture of air with a controlled quantity of added oxygen is used for hyperinflation. Under most circumstances the use of 100% oxygen is unnecessary, and it may promote alveolar collapse following suction. The analgesic effect produced by a mixture of 50% nitrous oxide and 50% oxygen (Entonox) may be helpful when carrying out this treatment.

Analgesia

Some form of sedation is often necessary before treating the patient, or treatment can be timed to coincide with sedation already prescribed.

VARIATIONS OF TREATMENT WITH SPECIFIC CONDITIONS

1 Post-cardiac surgery

The indication for treatment by manual hyperinflation with chest vibration depends

67

on the volume of bronchial secretions present, and also on the cardio-vascular state of the patient (p. 59).

If treatment is given during the first post-operative day, the patient should probably remain supine; while supporting the incision with one hand, gentle vibrations are given to the side of the chest with the other hand. The physiotherapist must be aware of any change in the ECG pattern, or colour of the patient. The blood pressure should be taken during treatment, if it has been unstable.

If the patient is treated in side-lying, and has had a median sternotomy, care must be taken to avoid giving too much pressure to the lateral chest wall. The hands are placed more posteriorly than laterally, and during suction the incision should be supported by one hand and forearm, while vibrating the posterior aspect of the chest wall with the other hand.

2 Post-cardiac surgery in infants

The same type of treatment can be used for infants if it is indicated. A small bag ($\frac{1}{2}$-litre capacity) is used for inflation; it must be carefully controlled as it is very easy to over-inflate an infant's lungs, so causing a pneumothorax.

Saline (0·5 ml for a small baby) can be instilled before manual inflation. If it is inserted into the top of the endotracheal (or tracheostomy) tube, very little will reach the bronchi because of the small volume. It is more effective to fill a catheter with saline and, leaving the syringe attached, insert it into the endotracheal tube as far as it will go, withdraw it 1 cm (to ensure that it is above the carina), and then instil a further 0·5 ml of saline.

An infant's airways are so narrow that a small amount of mucus can block off a large area of lung tissue and rapid deterioration in the patient's condition may occur. Efficient, quick and regular suction is essential for any infant nursed on a ventilator.

3 Post-pulmonary surgery

If a patient requires IPPV following pulmonary surgery, physiotherapy with manual hyperinflation may be helpful. It can, if necessary, be combined with postural drainage for the appropriate area. It may be contra-indicated if there is an air leak, or any sign of surgical emphysema.

4 Acute exacerbations of chronic bronchitis

There are generally copious thick secretions in the lung bases of patients with chronic bronchitis who require intubation and ventilation. Initially, vigorous physiotherapy will be needed at least every two hours. The patient can be positioned for drainage of the affected lobes before and during treatment. The chest shaking can be more energetic than with surgical patients, as there is no painful incision.

5 Asthma

Occasionally a patient suffering from asthma may be intubated and ventilated. The small airways may be plugged with bronchial casts, and when the secretions start to liquefy, physiotherapy, consisting of hyperinflation and chest vibrations, may be required. Some physicians will order up to 10 ml of normal saline solution to be instilled before physiotherapy, to assist in loosening these casts. As bronchospasm may make manual hyperinflation very difficult, and the spasm may be aggravated by the chest vibrations, it is often helpful to give a bronchodilator before treatment. If the patient has severe bronchospasm and the secretions have not liquefied, treatment should be withheld.

6 Respiratory muscle paralysis

If the respiratory muscles are paralysed, for example by acute polyneuritis or poliomyelitis, IPPV may be necessary. Manual hyperinflation is a suitable method of treatment, but 'rib springing' is often a more effective means of moving the secretions than chest vibrations in the paralysed patient.

7 Tetanus

Severe cases of tetanus may be therapeutically paralysed and nursed on a ventilator. The treatment is similar to that for paralysed patients, but since there is no cough reflex, and often a hypersecretion from the bronchial mucosa, frequent turning and accurate positioning of the chest are essential to maintain clear airways.

8 Crushed chest

If a patient with a crushed chest requires IPPV, chest shaking to the affected side is usually contra-indicated. Positioning of the patient, combined with manual hyperinflation, may be given if there is no air leak. Positions may need to be modified if multiple injuries have been sustained. During suction and coughing, the chest should be supported firmly by the physiotherapist.

Contra-indications

1 Hyperinflation with chest vibrations can, in some cases, produce a fall in cardiac output, and a lowering of the arterial oxygen tension. It should never be undertaken unless there is some valid indication. Medical advice must always be sought before undertaking this form of treatment.

2 If a patient is suffering from acute pulmonary oedema, physiotherapy is contra-indicated. The pulmonary oedema can be increased by tracheal suction, and chest vibrations may also act as an irritant. The proximal secretions are removed by suction when necessary. Physiotherapy should be postponed until medical treatment has controlled the situation.

3 If there is a pneumothorax, surgical emphysema, or an intercostal tube in place to control an air leak, hyperinflation is likely to be contra-indicated.

Alternative method of chest treatment

If hyperinflation is contra-indicated, but physiotherapy is required to assist removal of secretions, an alternative method may be used. The chest is vibrated in time with the expiratory phase of the ventilator instead of giving any extra inflation. The patient can be positioned, saline instilled, and suction and coughing performed in exactly the same way as previously described.

Limb movements

Unconscious or paralysed patients should have passive movements to all their limbs. Active movements should be encouraged whenever possible.

For patients with neurological conditions, the basic principles for positioning, nursing and subsequent rehabilitation should be applied.

'Weaning' from a ventilator

'Weaning' from the ventilator is started when the patient's condition has improved sufficiently, and should be carried out under the supervision of the anaesthetist. The patient may start by breathing without the ventilator for short periods, and the length of time is increased according to the anaesthetist's instructions. The respiratory and pulse rates are recorded during spontaneous breathing, and blood gas measurements are made intermittently. If there are signs of respiratory distress, the anaesthetist is informed, and the patient is reconnected to the ventilator.

For patients breathing independently through a tracheostomy tube, humidification is essential to prevent bronchial secretions becoming thick and tenacious. An attachment to the tracheostomy tube will provide humidified air with the appropriate amount of additional oxygen.

Breathing exercises should be started during this stage to re-educate active use of the diaphragm and lateral basal chest movements. The patient should be encouraged to cough actively, instead of relying entirely on the stimulation of the suction cathether.

When the patient is breathing independently for several hours in the day, the physiotherapy would probably comprise active breathing exercises in the side-lying position with vibrations, active coughing and tracheal suction. Manual hyperinflation can be continued if necessary, but this should be stopped as soon as the patient is able to cough effectively, so that he can manage without assistance once the tube has been removed.

After removal of the tube, the dressing covering the tracheostomy should be as airtight as possible, but it is still necessary to teach the patient to hold the site of the tracheostomy firmly while coughing (fig. 49); otherwise some of the secretions and air are blown out through the incision instead of being expectorated from the mouth, and the full force of the cough is wasted.

For the first forty-eight hours after removal of a tracheostomy tube, it is often necessary to increase the frequency of treatments to assist clearance of secretions. At this stage, the assistance of IPPB (Intermittent Positive Pressure Breathing) with physiotherapy may help the patient to overcome what may be a critical period (p. 71).

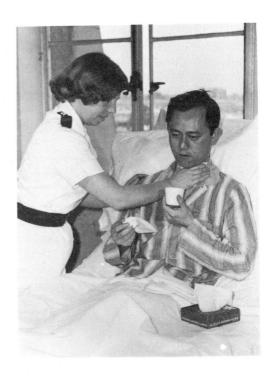

Fig. 49. *Coughing after removal of tracheostomy tube. By courtesy of Dr I.C.W. English.*

BRONCHIAL LAVAGE

When there is a tenacious exudate in the periphery of the lungs, either in the terminal bronchioles or alveoli, which is not responsive to the routine methods of removal (e.g. coughing and postural drainage), the procedure known as bronchial lavage is occasionally used. It is indicated in such conditions as intractable attacks of asthma and alveolar proteinosis. If the exudate in the periphery of the lungs is allowed to remain, it impairs aeration of the alveoli and inhibits gas transfer.

The aim of bronchial lavage is to flush out as much of the exudate as possible. It is a skilled procedure carried out under general anaesthesia using a double lumen tube. Approximately one litre of a warmed electrolyte solution with a physiological pH is instilled temporarily into one lung; after remaining a few minutes in the lung, the fluid is drained out by varying the position of the patient and by suction on the appropriate lumen of the tube. The instillation and drainage of fluid is usually repeated several times.

The physiotherapist may be requested to assist drainage of the fluid from the lung by two methods: firstly, by chest shaking over the treated lung which is co-ordinated with inflation of the other lung; a two-fold compression is thus exerted which assists expulsion of the fluid. Secondly, to remove the last remaining fluid, the more orthodox method of manual hyperinflation of the treated lung is used combined with chest shaking and postural drainage for all lobes.

Following the bronchial lavage, when the patient has regained consciousness, encouragement to cough will be necessary, and possibly postural drainage.

INTERMITTENT POSITIVE PRESSURE BREATHING (IPPB)

Use of an Intermittent Positive Pressure Breathing machine (IPPB) can be extremely valuable when chest physiotherapy alone is not having the desired effect. The ventilator can provide more effective aeration of the alveoli, and can promote expectoration; it is also a means of administering drugs and humidity directly into the airways. IPPB is most beneficial when it is used as an adjunct to physiotherapy; the maximum benefit is not achieved if a patient uses the machine without correct instruction.

There are several types of IPPB apparatus suitable for use with physiotherapy. At this hospital the 'Bird Mark 7' is employed, but others such as the 'Bennett T.V-4' or 'P.V-3P' are equally efficient. These machines are pressure-cycled ventilators driven by compressed oxygen or air. Some other models are driven electrically.

The essential features of an IPPB apparatus for use with physiotherapy are:

1 *Positive pressure* range of at least 0–30 cm H_2O.

2 *Simplicity* of controls.

3 *Portability*: the apparatus should be compact and easily movable from patient to patient.

4 *Sensitivity*: the inspiratory phase should be initiated ('triggered') by the patient with minimal effort. Fully automatic control is unpleasant for most patients and unnecessary for physiotherapy, but a hand triggering device is a useful asset on occasions.

5 *Flow control*: in machines such as the 'Bird Mark 7' the inspiratory gas is delivered at a flow rate which can be pre-set by means of a control knob. Optimal distribution of gas is achieved at relatively slow flow rates.

However, if the patient is very short of breath and has a fast respiratory rate, a slow inspiratory period may be unacceptable. It will then be necessary to deliver the gas initially at a fast rate. It is important to have the facility for adjusting the flow rate to suit the individual patient.

On other machines such as the 'Bennett' there is no adjustment necessary as an automatic variable flow is provided. This is called 'flow sensitivity' and means that the flow of inspired gas adapts to the resistance of the individual patient's airways.

6 *Nebuliser*: an efficient device for nebulisation is essential. The machine must never deliver unhumidified gas. In order to provide an effective means of administering drugs the nebuliser must be capable of producing fine particles, and of delivering the contents quickly (3–4 ml in 10 minutes). A large nebuliser (500 ml) can be fitted into the circuit if frequent and prolonged use of the ventilator is required.

7 *'Air-mix' control*: if the machine is driven by oxygen it is necessary that air is entrained in order to deliver a mixture of air and oxygen. 100% oxygen should never be delivered to the patient. Ideally the machine should be driven by compressed air and a controlled quantity of oxygen added according to the patient's requirements (p. 16). With the 'Bird Mark 7', a simple method of achieving a 24–25% oxygen concentration is to run 2 litres of oxygen through a hypodermic needle into the inlet port of the micronebuliser, the machine being driven by compressed air.

8 *Mouthpiece or mask*: the majority of patients prefer to use a mouthpiece for IPPB, but a face mask is essential for treatment of confused patients.

9 *Breathing-head assembly*: it is most economical to have several sets for each IPPB machine. A breathing-head assembly consists of a mouthpiece or mask, exhalation valve, micro-nebuliser with tubing, and two channel tubing which connects the former parts to the machine.

To prevent cross infection, it is essential for each patient to have a complete breathing-head assembly which is sterilised at least every week or when the course of treatment is completed. The machine itself can be moved from patient to patient.

Preparation for treatment

1 The nebuliser is filled with the required solution. Any drug used in the nebuliser must be prescribed by the physician or surgeon in charge of the patient.

The bronchodilator commonly used is a 0·5% solution of Salbutamol (Ventolin). To give a dose of 2·5 mg, 0·5 ml of Salbutamol is combined with 3 ml of normal saline. Normal saline solution alone may be used for humidification. Some physicians prescribe acetyl cysteine ('Airbron') but in this case the machine must be driven by air as oxygen renders the substance less effective. Glycerols are unsuitable for some nebulisers.

2 The breathing-head assembly is connected to the ventilator, and the ventilator is connected to the driving gas.

3 The physiotherapist must ensure that the 'air-mix' control is in position for the entrainment of air.

4 If the machine has an 'expiratory timer' (automatic control), this is turned off.

5 The controls of the ventilator are set. With the 'Bird Mark 7' an average setting is: pressure at 15, flow rate at 7, and sensitivity at 7. These settings are varied according to each individual's requirements. It is sometimes easiest to start with these three controls set at 10, and to adjust them after the

patient has become accustomed to using the ventilator. The pressure and nebuliser are the only controls to be set on the 'Bennett'.

6 The ventilator is turned on to ensure that the nebuliser is functioning correctly, and that there are no leaks in the breathing-head assembly.

Treatment of the patient

The position of the patient depends on the condition for which the IPPB is being given; it may be effectively used in the sitting, high side-lying, or side-lying positions (figs. 50 and 51). The patient should be comfortable and able to relax the upper chest and shoulder girdle.

The patient should be told to close his lips firmly round the mouthpiece and to breathe in through his mouth; he will then feel the ventilator start to 'blow air' into his chest and he should relax and try not to breathe out against this. If he does exhale before the ventilator cycles into expiration, the needle on the pressure gauge swings round to a much higher pressure than that set, indicating incorrect performance.

When using the mouthpiece, it is often necessary to use a nose-clip until the patient becomes accustomed to the ventilator. Without this, there is a tendency to allow air to leak through the nose, and as a result the ventilator will not reach the required pressure and will not cycle into expiration. This same problem arises if the patient does not close his lips firmly around the mouthpiece, or when using a mask if it is not held firmly enough to produce an air-tight seal with the face.

After a few breaths have been taken using the ventilator correctly, the patient is encouraged to use the lower chest during treatment. The physiotherapist places her fingers on the chest as for diaphragmatic

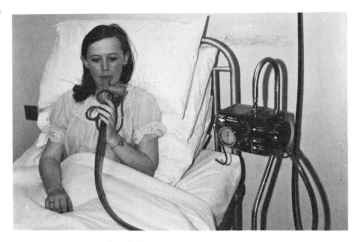

Fig. 50. *IPPB in sitting.*

breathing; basal expansion can also be encouraged.

Expiration should be quiet and relaxed. Forced expiration with or without IPPB tends to increase airways obstruction (p. 6).

The exhalation valve may be provided with a retard cap which can be used to give resistance to expiration. Unless it is specifically ordered, it is preferable to remove this cap, as it can easily be placed in the wrong position and impede expiration.

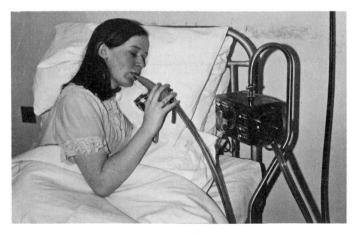

Fig. 51. *IPPB in high side-lying.*

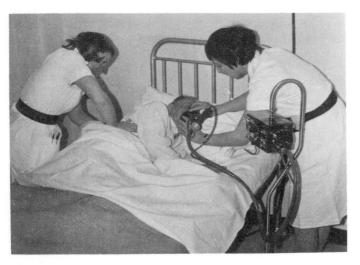

Fig. 52. *IPPB with mask.*

To avoid hyperventilation and resultant dizziness, the patient should pause momentarily after expiration, before the next inspiration.

Treatment continues until the contents of the nebuliser are used. This takes approximately 15 minutes.

INDICATIONS FOR USE OF IPPB

1 Relief of bronchospasm

A patient with severe bronchospasm may obtain relief from administration of a bronchodilator (e.g. Salbutamol) by means of IPPB. If bronchial secretions are also present, the bronchodilator should be given in a comfortable relaxed position (high side-lying or half-lying), and physiotherapy to assist the removal of secretions should not be attempted until the bronchodilator has taken effect.

To estimate the effect of the treatment, it is helpful to record the FEV$_1$ or peak expiratory flow rate before and after treatment.

The physician must prescribe the bronchodilator and the frequency with which it is to be given. If treatment is required frequently (e.g. every hour or two hours) it may be necessary to use normal saline solution for alternate treatments.

2 Acute exacerbation of chronic bronchitis

For patients in respiratory failure due to sputum retention, which may occur during an acute exacerbation of chronic bronchitis, treatment with IPPB can be invaluable and intubation avoided (p. 27).

The patient is often confused, drowsy, and unable to cough effectively. With this type of patient it is often necessary to use the mask, and it is helpful to have another physiotherapist or a nurse to assist with the treatment (figs. 52 and 53). If possible, the patient should be turned on to his side and the foot of the bed elevated. One physiotherapist, or the nurse, should elevate the jaw and hold the mask firmly over the patient's face ensuring an air-tight fit, whilst the other physiotherapist shakes the chest on expiration. The operator holding the mask may use the manual control on the machine in order to impose effective deep breaths on the patient. It may be necessary to continue this treatment for up to half an hour initially, the patient often becoming more rational after about the first ten minutes and starting to cough effectively. If effective coughing is not stimulated, naso-tracheal suction may be necessary.

At first, treatment should be given for fifteen to thirty minutes and be repeated at hourly or two-hourly intervals. As the patient's condition improves the frequency of treatments is reduced.

If the machine is driven by oxygen, the

physiotherapist should watch particularly for any increase in drowsiness during treatment. Compressed air is sometimes recommended for these patients (p. 18).

3 Sputum retention in medical and surgical conditions

In conditions such as bronchitis or a chest infection secondary to emphysema, or in post-operative cases, the patient may breathe and cough ineffectively and retain sputum. IPPB assists the physiotherapist by giving humidity with the nebuliser, and aerating the lungs more effectively, thus helping to mobilise secretions. Normal saline is used in the nebuliser unless bronchospasm is also present, and the treatment is carried out in conjunction with postural drainage. Bronchoscopy may be avoided if the sputum can be cleared. Possibly only one or two IPPB treatments will be necessary. As soon as the patient can breathe deeply enough to loosen secretions and cough effectively, physiotherapy alone is continued.

4 Following cardiac surgery

If a patient is suffering from pulmonary dysfunction after heart surgery (p. 62), or is too tired to carry out breathing exercises efficiently, IPPB may be used to increase the tidal volume. Localised basal expansion exercises are given in conjunction to improve alveolar ventilation.

5 Laryngeal dysfunction and phrenic nerve paralysis

Occasionally the larynx is traumatised if an endotracheal tube is in place for several days. If resection of the left recurrent laryngeal nerve is necessary during radical pneumonectomy, there is difficulty in closure

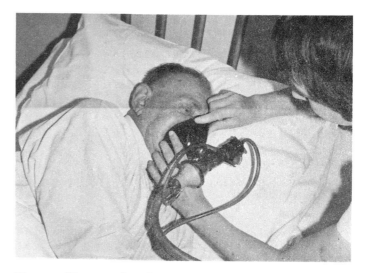

Fig. 53. *Close-up of mask.*

of the vocal cords. In both instances IPPB is found to be helpful in assisting ventilation and removal of secretions.

If the phrenic nerve has been divided during pneumonectomy (p. 51), IPPB may be necessary to assist ventilation postoperatively. The surgeon must give his permission.

6 Closure of tracheostomy

During the period of healing of a tracheostomy after 'weaning' from a ventilator, the patient may become easily fatigued and unable to clear the airways adequately. IPPB with physiotherapy may help the patient surmount this difficult period. In order for the machine to function correctly, it is often necessary to hold the tracheostomy dressing firmly to prevent any air-leak.

7 Chest deformity

Patients who have chest wall deformity and respiratory muscle weakness, such as may occur after acute poliomyelitis, are likely to have a reduced vital capacity. During chest infections, assistance will be needed to clear the airways. If the rib cage is rigid, a higher pressure setting on the IPPB machine is necessary to produce adequate ventilation.

8 Brain damage

The patient with brain damage may be unable to co-operate with the physiotherapist in maintaining clear airways. IPPB with the face mask to provide periods of effective ventilation, combined with chest vibrations, may be indicated.

9 Re-education of paralysed patients

IPPB machines with a sensitivity control can be used in the re-education of paralysed respiratory muscles, e.g. following acute polyneuritis. The sensitivity control is initially set at a low figure, and then gradually increased to necessitate greater inspiratory effort. In this way the machine may be used to 'wean' patients from non-triggered positive pressure ventilators.

10 Re-education of breathing pattern

Patients with severe emphysema or chronic bronchitis find difficulty in performing normal basal chest movement. A paradoxical movement of the lower rib cage often develops (p. 26). IPPB with resistance of the physiotherapist's hands over the lower ribs, can assist in re-education of some lateral basal movement of the rib cage.

11 Administration of antibiotics

In occasional cases of resistant chest infection, inhalations of antibiotics are prescribed, and can be delivered from an IPPB nebuliser. The nebuliser should be thoroughly washed and the jets probed immediately after use, as these substances are sticky and can block the nebuliser. If the patient is having physiotherapy to assist removal of secretions, this should be given before the inhalation of antibiotic.

12 Home use

A very small percentage of patients with chronic respiratory disease require an IPPB machine at home. If it is considered that by using a machine at home, the patient will avoid admissions to hospital, it may be justified for the hospital or patient to buy one. An electrically operated ventilator is usually more convenient at home unless the patient needs additional oxygen.

CONTRA-INDICATIONS TO IPPB

1 Pneumothorax

IPPB would tend to increase a pneumothorax and should therefore not be used.

2 Haemoptysis

3 Post-operative air leaks

A patient with an intercostal drain to control an air leak, who also has sputum retention, should only use IPPB with the surgeon's permission. The pressure should be kept low (no higher than 13 cm H_2O).

4 Cystic fibrosis

Patients with cystic fibrosis have a tendency

to pneumothoraces. IPPB should only be used at the request of the physician, and the pressure should be kept low.

5 Unnecessary use

If a patient can breathe and cough adequately without IPPB, or no longer requires a bronchodilator, it is a waste of time and apparatus to give treatment with IPPB.

6 Addiction to IPPB

IPPB apparatus is expensive. It is unwise to allow patients to become dependent on the machine if it is not essential. Patients should be 'weaned' from the machine as soon as it is no longer serving a genuine purpose.

Sterilisation of equipment

Each patient should have his own breathing-head assembly so that the risks of cross infection are minimised.

After each treatment the mouthpiece is scrubbed with soap and warm water, and the nebuliser is rinsed and dried. The tubing is detached from the ventilator and the complete assembly stored in a polythene bag or other suitable container until required again. After the course of treatment the entire breathing-head assembly is sterilised.

To sterilise the breathing-head assembly, the mouthpiece is scrubbed, and the other component parts are disassembled and rinsed; the capillary jets or tubing of the nebuliser are cleaned with the probe provided for the purpose. The separate pieces are then immersed in a suitable disinfectant for the prescribed length of time. (Cidex may be used. Hibitane and Phenol are not suitable for this equipment.) They are then rinsed thoroughly with water to eliminate the taste of the disinfectant. A syringe should be used to flush the capillary tubing. Finally, the equipment is dried, reassembled, and stored in a suitable container until required again.

If there is a shortage of equipment, the complete breathing-head assembly must be sterilized between each patient's treatment. It is not adequate to sterilise only the mouthpiece and exhalation valve.

The ventilator itself is sterilised with ethylene oxide gas.

A machine used for a patient with particularly resistant strains of bacteria, should if possible be confined to that patient. It should then be sterilised before use on any other patient.

Servicing of equipment

The IPPB machine should be cleaned internally and overhauled every three months by a specialist engineer.

It is important to keep a stock of spare parts so that any perishable or breakable parts such as rubber washers or springs can be replaced quickly.

Index

The Brompton Hospital Guide to Chest Physiotherapy

Second Edition, Third Printing

£1.75 net

This little book is derived from *Physiotherapy for Medical and Surgical Thoracic Conditions* originally compiled at Brompton Hospital in 1960. Physiotherapy at the hospital was started in 1934 by Winifred Linton F.C.S.P. The techniques have been developed and modified by her successors in order to keep pace with advances in medicine and surgery. This new publication is completely rewritten and expanded to give a more comprehensive picture of physiotherapy in this field.

'Intended primarily for physiotherapists both student and trained, this book will be of immense value to all nurses, medical students and others working in this field.' *Nursing Times*

'This book is an excellent source of reference for students, nurses and qualified physiotherapists.' *Physiotherapy*

'I am sure this book will be in constant use in many schools of physiotherapy, cardiothoracic units, medical respiratory units and also read by others concerned with the respiratory patient.' *British Journal of Diseases of the Chest*

'This book is primarily a practical guide for physiotherapists. But anyone concerned with the treatment of chest conditions can profit from reading it.' *Tubercle*

Other titles of related interest

Respiratory Physiology: the Essentials
John B. West M.D. PH.D. 1974. 196 pages, 92 illustrations. Paper, £3.50

Respiratory Illness in Children
Howard E. Williams M.D. F.R.A.C.P. and Peter D. Phelan B.SC. M.D. F.R.A.C.P. May 1975. 384 pages, 123 illustrations. About £9.00

Lecture Notes on Respiratory Diseases
R. A. L. Brewis M.D. F.R.C.P. Summer 1975. 224 pages, 70 illustrations. Paper, about £4.00

Respiratory Diseases
John Crofton M.A. M.D. F.R.C.P. and Andrew Douglas M.B. CH.B. F.R.C.P. *Second Edition*, Summer 1975. 912 pages, 120 illustrations. About £15.00

Disorders of the Respiratory System
Gordon Cumming B.SC. PH.D. D.SC. M.B. CH.B. F.R.C.P. F.R.I.C. and Stephen J. Semple M.D. M.B.B.S. F.R.C.P. 1973. 576 pages, 80 illustrations. Cloth £9.90, limp £6.50

Lung Function: Assessment and Application in Medicine
J. E. Cotes D.M.(Oxon) M.R.C.P.(Lond.). *Third Edition*, 1975. 640 pages, 120 illustrations. £13.00

Respiratory Failure
M. K. Sykes M.A. M.B. B.CHIR. D.A. F.F.A.R.C.S., M. W. McNicol M.B. M.R.C.P. and E. J. M. Campbell B.SC. PH.D. M.D. F.R.C.P. 1969 (*Reprinted* 1970, 1971). 382 pages, 69 illustrations. £2.75

Pulmonary Physiology in Clinical Practice
William R. Pace Jr M.D. *Second Edition*, 1970. 186 pages, 54 illustrations. £2.15

Spinal Cord Injuries: Comprehensive Management and Research
Sir Ludwig Guttman C.B.E. O.ST.J. M.D. F.R.C.P. F.R.C.S. HON.D.SC.(LIV.) HON.D.CHIR.(DURHAM) HON.LI.D.(DUBLIN). 1973. 712 pages, 273 illustrations. £16.00

The Lung in Health and Disease
Charles F. Geschickter M.D. 1973. 208 pages, 85 illustrations. Lippincott, paper £4.95

BLACKWELL SCIENTIFIC PUBLICATIONS

OXFORD LONDON EDINBURGH MELBOURNE

ISBN 0 632 09670 5